ANTIBIOTIC PROPHYLAXIS IN SURGERY

John E. Conte, Jr., M.D.

Associate Professor, Departments of Medicine and Microbiology;
Chief, Division of Infectious Diseases,
University of California, – San Francisco
San Francisco, California

Leonard S. Jacob, M.D., Ph.D.

Research Associate Professor of Pharmacology,
Medical College of Pennsylvania;
Vice President, Clinical Research and Development
(North America),
Smith Kline & French Laboratories,
Philadelphia, Pennsylvania

Hiram C. Polk, Jr., M.D.

Professor and Chairman, Department of Surgery
University of Louisville School of Medicine,
Louisville, Kentucky

EDITH SCHWAGER   *Executive Editor*

ANTIBIOTIC PROPHYLAXIS IN SURGERY

A Comprehensive Review

 J. B. Lippincott Company
Philadelphia
London   Mexico City   New York
St. Louis   São Paulo   Sydney

Acquisitions Editor: Micaela Palumbo
Sponsoring Editor: Sanford J. Robinson
Manuscript Editor: Delois Patterson
Indexer: Julie Schwager
Art Director: Maria S. Karkucinski
Designer: Susan A. Caldwell
Production Supervisor: N. Carol Kerr
Compositor: Publisher's Network
Printer/Binder: R.R. Donnelley & Sons Company

The authors and publisher have exerted every effort to ensure that drug
selection and dosage set forth in this text are in accord with current recommendations and practice at the time of publication. However, in view of
ongoing research, changes in government regulations, and the constant flow
of information relating to drug therapy and drug reactions, the reader is urged
to check the package insert for each drug for any change in indications and
dosage and for added warnings and precautions. This is particularly important
when the recommended agent is a new or infrequently employed drug.

1   3   5   6   4   2

Library of Congress Cataloging in Publication Data

Conte, John E., Jr.
  Antibiotic prophylaxis in surgery.
  Bibliography.
  Includes index.
  1. Surgical wound infections—Prevention.
2. Antibiotics. I. Jacob, Leonard S. II. Polk, Hiram C.,Jr.
1936-   . III. Title. [DNLM: 1. Antibiotics—
Therapeutic Use. 2. Surgical wound infection—Preven-
tion and control. WO 185 C761a]
RD98.3.C66 1984   617'.22   84-888
ISBN 0-397-50671-6

PREFACE

This book is intended to provide surgeons, internists, house staff, hospital pharmacists, and medical students with a reference and up-to-date guide to the use of antibiotic prophylaxis in surgery. the chapters are organized uniformly. After a brief introduction, which is usually historical, the clinical, microbiologic, and pharmacokinetic aspects of prophylaxis are discussed. Each chapter also contains a comprehensive review of the literature in that surgical subspecialty, followed by practical recommendations. In some areas of surgery, controlled trials have validated the usefulness of antibiotic prophylaxis in certain situations, whereas in other areas (such as neurosurgery), we express our opinions based on our best judgment, given the evidence that is available.

Chapter 10, Obstetrics and Gynecology, was written by Ronald S. Gibbs, M.D., University of Texas Health Science Center, San Antonio.

The use of antibiotic prophylaxis in surgery is surrounded by controversy, perhaps more than many other areas in medicine. Clinical practice has evolved from empiric, often prolonged antibiotic regimens to more standard protocols, usually with short-term perioperative prophylaxis. We now have a much clearer understanding of the risk of infection associated with different surgical procedures and the clinical characteristics that might aggravate or mitigate those risks. Thus, in procedures with notoriously high infection rates, antibiotic prophylaxis is useful. In procedures with low infection rates, the benefits of prophylaxis may be questionable. An exception to this rule of thumb is the implantation of prosthetic devices or materials, as in orthopedic, vascular, or cardiac surgery. Although infection rates are low in these "clean" procedures, the consequences of infection in the operated site are potentially devastating. Thus prophylaxis is justified and recommended in these situations.

We believe that the historical controversy attending antibiotic prophylaxis in surgery has given way to guidelines derived from controlled clinical trials. Many patients will benefit from a short course of perioperative (or perhaps single-dose) prophylaxis in certain surgical procedures.

John E. Conte, Jr., M.D.
Leonard S. Jacob, M.D., Ph.D
Hiram C. Polk, Jr., M.D.

ACKNOWLEDGMENTS

We gratefully acknowledge the invaluable assistance of Ms. Karen Mah-Hing in preparing the manuscript.

Our sincere thanks to Mrs. Patricia Bensinger and Mrs. Shirley Cook for their expert secretarial help.

CONTENTS

ANTIBIOTIC PROPHYLAXIS IN SURGERY

Chapter **1**

HISTORICAL AND CLINICAL CONSIDERATIONS

HISTORICAL CONSIDERATIONS

It is helpful to differentiate semantically between prophylaxis and early therapy. *Prophylaxis* in its purest sense implies administration of the putative agent before bacterial contamination occurs, e.g., before an elective colon resection. *Early therapy* best connotes immediate, or at least prompt, institution of therapy as soon as the patient is seen or the diagnosis is made; usually contamination or infection (or both) will have preceded the initiation of therapy. This situation is exemplified by perforative appendicitis when administration of antibiotics is begun as soon as the diagnosis is made but, by definition, after bacterial contamination has occurred.

The patient with nonperforative appendicitis is a perfect example of this semantic paradox. Antibiotics begun before appendectomy may be considered therapeutic with respect to appendiceal disease and at the same time prophylactic with respect to prevention of infection in the operative incision that will be used to remove the appendix. Whether therapy, prophylaxis or anticipatory therapy, the issue at hand is the timely and wise administration of antibiotics.

Sulfonamides became available for clinical use in the late 1930s. In 1939, Jensen et al.[1] described their experience with the prophylactic use of topical sulfanilamide in open fractures. Using historical data from their institution, they concluded that sulfanilamide used prophylactically in open fractures had decreased the incidence of postoperative infection from 27% to less than 5%. In their series of 39 patients with compound fractures or dislocations, there was no primary wound infection. This report ushered in more than four decades of controversy, which still persists, over the prophylactic use of antibiotics in surgery.

In 1945, Meleney[2] published the results of a national cooperative study of the use of sulfonamides, topically and systemically, to prevent infection in civilian traumatic injuries. This monumental effort, which involved nine participating hospitals and 2,191 patients, had important implications for the management of war-related injuries. Almost in despair, the author concluded:

> It was hoped that it would be possible to demonstrate by statistical methods that the sulfonamides were capable of materially reducing the incidence of infection in wounds treated under the conditions to be found in a number of good civilian hospitals. In fact, it was not beyond the hope of certain individuals that they would be able to do this in spite of certain compromises with surgical principles such as incomplete removal of devitalized tissue and gross contamination—such as might be necessary under the stress of military conditions or when careless ward dressings are done without due regard to the possibilities of secondary wound contamination from the hands or from the noses and throats of the attendants. But such was not the case. Our carefully analyzed figures show that when the local conditions favored infection, the controls on the whole did better than the drug-treated cases. These are precisely the conditions in which it was hoped that the drugs might be of value. This tends to lend weight to the belief that the presence of devitalized or damaged tissue in some way inhibits the bacteriostatic action of the sulfonamides.

Penicillin was used for the first time in the United States in 1942 to treat a woman who was suffering post partum from β-hemolytic streptococcal sepsis.[3] The response was dramatic and the therapy life-saving. Perhaps because of this initial favorable therapeutic experience, attempts were made in the late 1940s and early 1950s to evaluate the effectiveness of prophylactic penicillin in various kinds of gynecologic and obstetric surgery.[4-7] These investigators concluded that, in general, prophylaxis was of value.

By the late 1940s and early 1950s, streptomycin and tetracycline were widely available. Reports[8] of their prophylactic use appeared shortly after their introduction. Guilbeau et al.[9] described the marked effect of chlortetracycline on the bacterial flora of the normal or the infected postpartum uterus. These investigators also administered a tetracycline prophylactically to parturient women and concluded that febrile morbidity was reduced.

Early emphasis was placed on the use of antibiotic prophylaxis in obstetrics and gynecology and for burns and other trauma. However, reports of prophylactic antibiotic use in prostatectomy and appendectomy also appeared in the late 1940s.[10,11]

In 1946, Prince[10] reported the use of sulfadiazine and penicillin prophylactically for transurethral resection of the prostate. Thirty-six patients were given sulfadiazine, 2 g, as a loading dose, followed by 1 g every 6 hours beginning the evening before surgery, and then penicillin, 20,000 units every 3 hours, beginning the morning of surgery. The drugs were continued until the catheter was removed postoperatively. Of 36 patients so treated, 17 were discharged from the hospital with sterile urine. Nineteen patients had positive urine cultures after operation, 8 of which contained *Pseudomonas* sp. and only one specimen had contained *Pseudomonas* sp. preoperatively. This was an early demonstration of the finding that antibiotics given prophylactically favor the emergence of resistant gram-negative rods.

Although a number of investigators demonstrated the effectiveness of sulfonamides[12,13] and penicillin[14,15] in the treatment of peritonitis in dogs and humans,[16] routine prophylactic administration of these drugs for appendectomy was not reported until 1947.[11] Using their routine therapy, except for the newly introduced use of penicillin and sulfadiazine, Griffin et al.[11] concluded that prophylactic administration of these drugs decreased the average hospital stay for patients with perforated appendices who underwent appendectomy from 19.6 days in 1935 (before this regimen) to 11.7 days in 1946 (after this regimen). Similarly, the mortality associated with appendectomy decreased from 7.6% for the years 1928 to 1932 to 0.9% in 1946.

By 1954, the practice of using antibiotic prophylaxis had become widespread, and warnings of the hazards of indiscriminate use began to appear. McKittrick and Wheelock[17] introduced a retrospective analysis of patients who had undergone abdominal surgery with the following statement:

> In recent years we have noted a widening utilization of the antibiotic agents in preparation for, or following routine surgical procedures. We have questioned the necessity, as well as the desirability, of dividing the responsibility for an elective surgical operation on the gastrointestinal tract between the technique of the surgeon and the chemotherapeutic or antibiotic agent. The increasing number of serious, even fatal, complications following the use of the antibiotics would seem to place upon us the responsibility of presenting evidence that the benefits to our patients from their routine use clearly outweigh the hazards,

and that the potential dangers against which they are supposed to protect cannot be avoided by careful surgical technique.

In their review of the effectiveness of prophylaxis with penicillin and streptomycin, the authors,[17] unable to demonstrate a favorable effect, concluded:

> One hundred and seventy-five patients with operations upon the gastrointestinal or biliary tracts were studied. This study failed to demonstrate benefits which are necessary to compensate for the discomforts, expense, and possible dangers associated with the prophylactic use of antibiotics following most elective operations on the gastrointestinal and biliary tracts.

However, as discussed later, antibiotic prophylaxis is effective in both colorectal and biliary tract surgery, under certain circumstances. McKittrick and Wheelock's study,[17] like many other retrospective ones, failed to appreciate the deleterious effect of initiating prophylaxis *after* operation. The basic experimental documentation[18] was not forthcoming until 3 years later, but it did provide a sound basis for the modern studies of systemic prophylaxis.

The use of antibiotic prophylaxis in numerous specialties and medical situations continued to proliferate. Their use was described, usually by retrospective review, in orthopedic surgery,[19] thoracic surgery, central nervous system surgery, oral surgery,[20] and vascular surgery.[21] As each new antibiotic became available, it was inevitably used in burn management, either topically or systemically, or both.

With the high rate of infection in burn injuries, it is not surprising that antibiotics were frequently used not only therapeutically but prophylactically. Finland et al.[22] found it difficult to determine whether sulfonamides administered only systemically prevented burn infection in victims of the Cocoanut Grove Nightclub (Boston) fire. However, Lyons,[23] who treated victims from the same fire at a different hospital, concluded that systemic sulfonamide and penicillin administration, or penicillin alone in some patients, was effective in controlling infection from burn wounds. The preponderant organisms reported subsequently in these patients were *Staphylococcus aureus,* β-hemolytic streptococci, and gram-negative rods.

Lowbury[24] and Taylor[25] reviewed the use of antibiotic prophylaxis in burns in Great Britain. Each believed that topical penicillin cream significantly reduced the number of burn infections caused by *Streptococcus pyogenes.* Both authors emphasized the emergence of *S. aureus* and gram-negative rods, particularly *Pseudomonas* sp., as important pathogens in burns.

Subsequently, Cason and Lowbury[26] reported the results of a controlled trial of topical neomycin-chlorhexidine-polymyxin (NCP) cream in burn patients. Colonization rates were reduced from 88% to 20% for *S. aureus* and from 24% to 5% for *S. pyogenes.* The cream was less effective in controlling *Pseudomonas* infection. These authors reported that systemic administration of chloramphenicol, tetracycline, erythromycin, and polymyxin were ineffective in preventing infection from burns, and emphasized the emergence of resistant organisms.

Altemeier et al.[27] retrospectively reviewed their experience with patients who had burn infections between 1942 and 1962. Several antibiotics were used prophylactically in 1,828 patients during that time (Table 1-1). These authors documented the evolution of gram-negative rods as the preponderant cause of burn wound infection.

Kefalides et al.,[28] in reviewing bacteriologic data on 314 burned children from 1957 to 1961, concluded that prophylaxis with various antibiotics available at that time "failed to prevent rapid colonization of burned areas and intestine by *Staph. aureus* and *Ps. aeruginosa.*"

A number of other authors voiced caution, emphasized the adverse effects of antibiotics on the normal flora, and described superinfection occurring during therapy.[29-33]

Smith[30] introduced his review with the following observations:

> Evidence is accumulating to show that the complex balance which exists among microörganisms constituting the normal flora of the body is disturbed by the prolonged administration of the newer antibiotics. This may result in the development of secondary vitamin deficiencies or the evolution of new infectious disease syndromes.
>
> The importance of the normal microbiologic flora in man was not appreciated until it was disorganized by the administration of the newer antibiotics. The basic phenomenon is not new, and biologists dealing with parasitic diseases of plants are familiar with the importance of the normal flora of the soil and its influence on the increase or decrease of the parasitic species.

Two years later, in 1954, Weinstein[31] reported on 68 superinfections occurring in 3,095 patients (2.2%) treated with one or more antibiotics between 1946 and 1953. Convincing evidence was presented relating superinfection to the location of primary infection, the type and duration of antibiotic therapy, and the patient's age. No correlation could be found between the type of organism causing the initial infection and the type of organism causing the superinfection.

Table 1–1. Chemotherapy and Prophylactic Antibiotic Therapy in the Management of 1,828 Burn Patients Treated Between January 1, 1942 and January 1, 1962

Antibiotic	1942-44 (%)	1951-53 (%)	1958-62 (%)
Sulfadiazine	27	—	—
Penicillin	0.7	100	86
Chloramphenicol	—	44	47
Oxytetracycline	—	27	18
Erythromycin	—	—	18
Streptomycin	—	1	13
Tetracycline	—	—	11
Polymyxin B	—	—	5
Novobiocin	—	—	4
Vancomycin	—	—	3

From Altemeier et al.,[27] with permission.

Indeed, antibiotics were promptly and widely used systemically to prevent infection in major burns. Although it was shown in 1960 (and it is generally held now) that penicillin prevents early streptococcal infection of superficial burns and donor sites in skin grafts, its influence on major sepsis and survival was not shown.[34] If anything, attempted prophylaxis in the burn patient tended to select resistant organisms, initially staphylococci, and promoted the shift from *Streptococcus* to *Staphylococcus* as the primary pathogen. Important work by Moncrief and Teplitz[35] on the pathology of the burn wound itself was crucial in interpreting these clinical efforts. The burn eschar is avascular, and they concluded that no amount of circulating antibiotic was likely to eradicate microbial invasion of literally thousands of grams of avascular eschar.

Virtually simultaneously and genuinely independently, Moncrief and his teacher, Moyer,[36] and their associates concluded that a sound approach would be to prevent microbial invasion by applying a topical "barrier," as it were, to the external surface of the avascular eschar. It had already been shown by Haynes et al.[37] that colonization was derived from the patient's enteric organisms and by environmental air-borne and contact-borne bacteria.

Lindberg et al.[38] applied mafenide hydrochloride, and Polk et al.[39] treated the wound with 0.5% aqueous silver nitrate; despite serious side effects with both methods, considerable improvement in the survival rate was noted immediately by both groups. These results denote the only statistically significant advance in survival of the badly burned patient since the advent of effective therapy for hypovolemic shock.[39]

In the 1960s differences of opinion continued to widen between internists and surgeons about surgical antibiotic prophylaxis. Antibiotics were frequently used by surgeons for all types of surgical procedures without regard to the risk of infection. They were usually administered postoperatively and for a prolonged time. Opponents argued that scientific proof of efficacy was lacking, that toxicity and the costs of antibiotic therapy exceeded the benefits, and that antibiotic prophylaxis had an adverse effect on the microbial flora.

The observations of Miles et al.[18] concerning the effective period of preventive antibiotic action in experimental lesions were an important step in understanding the rational use of surgical antibiotic prophylaxis. They demonstrated that antibiotics had to be present when an infective lesion originated, to achieve maximal prophylactic effect. Further, this "decisive period" ended after 3 hours. Interestingly, this is a property or characteristic of local infective lesions, and the "decisive period" applies to many other, non-antibiotic modifiers of local infection (Fig.1-1).

During the 1970s, an increasing number of studies on the use of antibiotic prophylaxis in surgery were undertaken. Chodak and

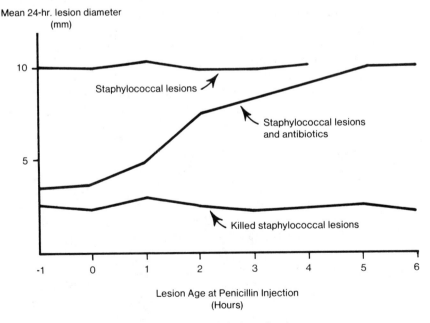

Fig. 1-1. Effective period of preventive antibiotic action in surgery.

Plaut,[40] however, found that only 24 of 131 articles met their criteria for appropriate design and hence generated evaluable data. DiPiro et al.[41] wrote a comprehensive review of English-language studies on surgical antimicrobial prophylaxis published between 1976 and 1980. These authors reviewed 76 "evaluable" reports, 57 of which demonstrated statistically significant decreases in infection rates resulting from the use of prophylactic antibiotics.

With this mounting evidence (although of variable quality) of effectiveness, surgical antibiotic prophylaxis for patients with a high risk of postoperative infection has been receiving greater acceptance. Indeed, the consensus of authoritative surgeons and experts in infectious diseases is that systemic antibiotic prophylaxis is generally a sound concept.[41-48]

PHARMACOLOGIC CONSIDERATIONS

Prophylactic antibiotic administration is the administration initially of an antibiotic or a combination of antibiotics to a patient who is asymptomatic or about to undergo operation. The antibiotic in this kind of situation is intended to prevent the development of infection. In medical situations, such as the prevention of meningococcal infection, prophylaxis may be instituted after exposure or, as in the prevention of rheumatic fever, prophylaxis may precede exposure. To prevent postoperative infection, antibiotics must always be administered before or at the beginning of the surgical procedure. Definitive antibiotic therapy refers to the administration of an antibiotic to treat an established infection; in contrast to empiric therapy, the organism usually has been identified by culturing, and its sensitivities have been determined.

The selection of an antibiotic for prophylaxis should be based on the site of potential infection and the microorganisms likely to be involved.[47] Appropriate guidelines for prophylaxis in surgery have evolved in a highly variable and irregular progression of studies. It is necessary to demonstrate that a group of patients is at significant risk of postoperative infectious complications. One must then determine that antibiotic prophylaxis has a statistically significant effect in reducing the incidence of these complications. It is also desirable to select the smallest dose of antibiotic that will be effective when given for the shortest period.[49]

Many studies that demonstrated a decrease in the rate of infections with prophylaxis have failed to show a decrease in overall mortality. This is not surprising *per se.* Potential advantages of prophylaxis include a decrease in mortality, morbidity, and financial expense as a consequence of preventing serious infections. The hazards and costs include allergic or toxic reactions to the drug, induced resistance of microbial flora, and the direct and indirect expense of the drug and its administration.[50]

Pharmacokinetics

The pharmacokinetics of the drugs considered for use must be reviewed to ensure adequate concentration at the site of the expected infection. Although there has been great progress in understanding many pharmacokinetic aspects of antibiotic use, such as peak serum levels, serum half-life, plasma and renal clearance, volume of distribution, and bioavailability, there has not been a concerted effort to use such knowledge systematically to improve the clinical results when antibiotics are used prophylactically. Application of such data should allow the surgeon to achieve maximal benefit from antimicrobial agents that are used preoperatively to prevent wound infection. As a matter of fact, wound antibiotic activity may be crucial in selecting an agent for systemic prophylaxis. The initial, rigidly controlled trial suggested this concept,[51] and additional data confirmed the point.[52] Indeed, the wound level of antibiotic activity and the duration of that level are essential for success.

Cephalothin is a slightly effective agent for prophylaxis. Its wound levels after a single 2-g dose are satisfactory, but antibiotic activity disappears from the surgical incision so quickly that little or no active drug is present at the time of wound closure 1½ to 3 hours later—times usually chosen for elective operations on the alimentary tract. Consistent with this concept is the recent simultaneous observation,[53] one in gynecologic operations and the other in colorectal surgery, that a single preoperative dose of a wound-active antibiotic may "lose" its effectiveness in operations lasting more than 2½ or 3 hours (personal communication from J.L. Sawyers, January 1983).

In the preventive use of antibiotics, one must weigh the potential benefits against possible deleterious side effects. Drug safety is vital. Although an antibiotic may have an extensive antibacterial spectrum in vitro, its pharmacologic properties may render it unsuitable in preventing infection in a particular area of the body. The antibiotic selected should have an antibacterial spectrum that includes the microorganisms most likely to cause postoperative infection at the surgical site. Particular attention to the resistance patterns of agents is needed and, ideally, the agent selected should have both gram-positive and gram-negative activity.[54]

The initial rapid fall in serum level following the parenteral administration of most antibiotics reflects their distribution in the body. This fall is followed by a more gradual decline that may be due to drug metabolism and renal or biliary excretion. The interstitial fluid and tissue drug concentrations are more important than the serum level. Tissue drug concentration, which can usually be determined, depends on the concentration gradient from serum to tissue. This gradient is determined by protein-binding, diffusibility, lipid solubility, molecular size, and pK values. Drugs usually reach higher levels in well-perfused lean tissues, such as the heart, lungs, or hepatorenal system, than in poorly perfused skin, bone, ligaments, or fat.[55]

The importance of serum protein-binding in the choice of an antibiotic is controversial. Tissue levels are not necessarily related to the degree of protein-binding. Cefazolin, which is more protein-binding than cephalothin, achieves higher tissue levels.[56] Since increased serum protein-binding may delay renal excretion, the net result will be high serum levels. If the dissociation constant of an antibiotic with a high degree of serum protein-binding is high, optimal tissue levels will be achieved and maintained.[56] Therefore, when antibiotics varying in serum protein-binding ability are compared, the agents with the highest values usually have the longest serum and tissue elimination half-lives, thus permitting less frequent administration.

The avidity (tightness of binding) of the antibiotic for serum proteins, as well as the more static concept of "percentage-bound," may affect both antibiotic kinetics and efficacy in treatment and prophylaxis. Further research is needed in this area.

Timing of Administration and Other Factors

The administration of antibiotics to prevent infective complications of surgery requires careful timing. Bacterial contamination most often occurs while the wound is open. This means that adequate serum and tissue levels must be achieved before the start of and during the operation. Intravenous administration results in a more rapid onset and higher serum levels, whereas intramuscular administration results in more sustained serum and tissue levels. It is now customary to administer prophylactic antibiotics on call to the operating room except in the case of cesarean section prophylaxis. Studies have shown short-term (less than 48 hours) perioperative prophylaxis to be as effective as prolonged antibiotic administration. Longer administration has no beneficial effect, either in theory or in practice; moreover, it may increase the risk of adverse effects and have a more profound effect on the bacterial flora, thereby encouraging overgrowth with more resistant organisms.[48]

The risk of infection, of course, depends on other factors besides the correct use of prophylactic antibiotics. The nature of the operation and the particular patient population undergoing surgery are important. It is universally agreed that there is no substitute for conscientious surgical technique. (See Appendix, which is a guideline for the control of surgical wound infection and is especially germane to matters other than antibiotics and their ultimate role.) This in itself may often achieve acceptable low infection rates without prophylaxis.

MICROBIOLOGIC CONSIDERATIONS

Table 1–2 lists the organisms most likely to cause postoperative infection, according to which part of the alimentary tract has been

Table 1–2. Organisms Most Commonly Causing Postoperative Infections in the Gastrointestinal Tract

Site	Aerobes	Anaerobes
Mouth and esophagus	Streptococci	Bacteroides (not *B. fragilis*), peptostreptococci, fusobacteria
Stomach	Enteric gram-negative bacilli, streptococci	Bacteroides (not *B. fragilis*), peptostreptococci, fusobacteria
Biliary tract	Enteric gram-negative bacilli, enterococci	Clostridia
Distal ileum and colon	Enteric gram-negative bacilli	*B. fragilis*, peptostreptococci, clostridia

Antibiotic Prophylaxis in Surgery

Table 1–3. Organisms Isolated from Wound Cultures at Massachusetts General Hospital in March 1976

Organism	Total Isolates	Total Significant Isolates*
Aerobic and facultative gram-positive bacteria	1,184	498
Aerobic and facultative gram-negative bacteria	504	262
Anaerobic bacteria	159	36
Fungi	66	27
Total	1,913	823

*Isolated in moderate or abundant amounts from primary culture.
From Moellering et al.,[49] with permission.

Table 1–4. Aerobic and Facultative Gram-Positive Bacteria Isolated From Wound Cultures at Massachusetts General Hospital in March 1976

Organism	Total Isolates	Total Significant Isolates*
Staphylococcus aureus	225	145
Staphylococcus epidermidis	374	106
Diphtheroids	149	86
Streptococci (excluding enterococci)	181	76
Enterococci	216	74
Micrococci	16	6
Lactobacillus sp.	6	2
Bacillus sp.	11	1
Staphylococcus sp.	4	1
Streptococcus pneumoniae	1	1
Listeria monocytogenes	1	0
Total	1,184	498

*Isolated in moderate or abundant amounts from primary culture.
From Moellering et al.,[49] with permission.

entered. Computer-facilitated analyses of the etiology of wound infection arising after various procedures provide a rational framework for the use of surgical antibiotic prophylaxis.[48] Table 1–3 summarizes all isolates from wound cultures during a 1-month period in one institution. As expected, the preponderant organisms (61% of significant isolates) were aerobic and facultative gram-positive bacteria. The second most common group of organisms (32% of significant isolates) was aerobic and facultative gram-negative bacteria; the third (4%) and the fourth (3%) were anaerobic bacteria and fungi, respectively. Tables 1–4 and 1–5 subcategorize the organisms listed in Table 1–3.

With reference to significant isolates, *S. aureus* and *Staphylococcus epidermidis* are the most common gram-positive bacteria, and *Escherichia coli*, *Pseudomonas aeruginosa*, and *Klebsiella pneumoniae* are the most common gram-negative bacteria. *Bacteroides fragilis* and *Candida albicans* are the preponderant anaerobes and yeast, respectively, isolated from wound cultures.

Most gram-negative and anaerobic wound infections occur after abdominal, pelvic, or trauma surgery. Staphylococci are the most common cause of postoperative wound infection associated with other types of surgery.

As discussed previously, patients with burn wound injuries are at high risk of infection. MacMillan[54] summarized the microbiologic causes of burn infection in 821 patients between 1970 and 1978 (Table 1–6).

Table 1–5. Aerobic and Facultative Gram-Negative Bacteria Isolated from Wound Cultures at Massachusetts General Hospital in March 1976

Organism	Total Isolates	Total Significant Isolates*
Escherichia coli	150	75
Pseudomonas aeruginosa	62	40
Klebsiella pneumoniae	68	35
Proteus mirabilis	50	24
Herellea vaginicola	37	17
Neisseria gonorrhoeae	15	12
Enterobacter cloacae	18	8
Haemophilus influenzae	9	8
Proteus morganii	12	5
Serratia marcescens	8	5
Klebsiella sp.	9	4
Neisseria sp.	7	4
Pseudomonas sp.	8	4
Enterobacter aerogenes	8	3
Alcaligenes sp.	3	2
Citrobacter freundii	5	2
Neisseria meningitidis	4	2
Citrobacter diversus	3	1
Proteus sp.	10	1
Others	18	10
Total	504	262

*Isolated in moderate or abundant amounts from primary culture.
From Moellering et al.,[49] with permission.

Table 1–6. Organisms Recovered From Burn Wounds in 821 Acute-Care Patients at Shriners Burn Institute (Cincinnati Unit)

Organism	Percentage of Patients From Whom Organisms Were Recovered in								
	1970	1971	1972	1973	1974	1975	1976	1977	1978
Staphylococcus aureus	70	65	65	70	75	80	85	78	68
β-hemolytic streptococci	8	3	8	8	3	3	5	13	10
Other streptococci	58	60	58	58	60	65	60	38	45
Pseudomonas aeruginosa	50	65	60	50	32	30	21	38	28
Klebsiella-Enterobacter	50	70	60	58	42	31	30	15	8
Escherichia coli	60	50	55	55	48	52	40	39	30
Proteus sp.	30	20	20	30	30	25	20	10	5
Other gram-negative organisms	50	35	40	30	25	23	20	25	32
Candida sp.	60	55	58	75	65	50	25	12	20
Candida albicans	35	40	45	62	55	35	40	24	18

From MacMillan,[54] with permission.

Although *S. aureus* is the most common pathogen isolated from burn wounds, one or more gram-negative rods are recovered from half of all burn wounds.

Many different organisms can cause postoperative infection depending on the clinical situation. The intelligent use of antibiotic prophylaxis must take into account the types and sensitivities of pathogens likely to be responsible for surgical infection.

SURGICAL CONSIDERATIONS

It is important to recognize that there are inherent risks of infections in wounds associated with intraabdominal surgery. In 1964 the Ad Hoc Committee of the Committee on Trauma of the National Research Council[57] promulgated a standard classification of surgical wounds, as follows:

CLASSIFICATION OF WOUNDS

Clean, Clean-Contaminated, Contaminated, and Dirty Wounds

The term *clean wound* applies to elective surgery with primary closure and no drain. The wound is nontraumatic and there is no inflammation. The gastrointestinal, respiratory, or urinary tract is not entered, and there is no break in aseptic technique. The anticipated infection rate in this category is less than 5%. In a large prospective study conducted by Cruse and Foord[58] of 36,382 clean wounds, only 624 (1.7%) became infected. Some groups recognize "refined-clean" as a separate class, exemplified by elective craniotomy rather than, for example, clean inguinal herniorrhaphy.

In *clean-contaminated* or *potentially contaminated* cases, a bacterially colonized viscus is entered without significant spillage or mechanical drainage. This category includes appendectomies and procedures involving entry into the vagina, the uninfected biliary tract, or the uninfected genitourinary tract. An infection rate of 10% to 20% is the consensus estimate for these surgical wounds; this rate is greatly influenced by patient and procedure mix. In a prospective study[58] of 7,335 clean-contaminated cases, 646 wound infections (8.8%) occurred.

The *contaminated* category includes cases in which acute inflammation (without pus formation) is encountered, or there is a major break in sterile technique, or gross spillage from the gastrointestinal tract occurs. The expected infection rate in contaminated cases is variously estimated to be between 16% and 40%. In the prospective study of Cruse and Foord,[58] of 2,613 contaminated wounds, there were 458 (17.5%) wound infections.

The category *dirty wounds* implies the presence of organisms in ordinarily sterile tissue before the operation and active infectious process. Included in this group are infections associated with traumatic wounds with retained devitalized tissue, foreign bodies, fecal contamination, delayed treatment, and wounds from a dirty source. This group also includes operations involving a perforated viscus and the presence of pus. The anticipated wound infection rate is greater than 30%. In Cruse and Foord's[58] prospective study of 1,586 such cases, 660 (41.6%) became infected.

This classification allows the surgeon to determine whether antimicrobial prophylaxis is appropriate for a specific procedure, a decision based on the risk of infection in that procedure weighed with a possible detrimental effect from antibiotic use. Since the wound infection rate for clean surgery is so low, the costs, both financial and ecologic, of antimicrobial prophylaxis probably exceed the benefits in most such instances. An exception is in those patients for whom infection is likely to be catastrophic. Examples of such situations include insertion of prostheses, such as cardiac valves, vascular grafts, and artificial joints, instances in which infection is so difficult to eradicate. Maintenance of low infection rates in clean cases is best obtained by strict adherence to principles of good surgical technique: gentle handling of tissue, de' bridement of devitalized tissue, adequate hemostasis, preservation of adequate blood supply, obliteration of dead spaces, absence of foreign body, and quick, painstaking technique.

Factors that have been shown to decrease the infection rate in clean cases include (1) a short preoperative stay in the hospital, (2) avoidance of shaving until just before operation, (3) minimizing the duration of surgery, and (4) a preoperative shower or bath with an antiseptic soap. Factors that are thought to increase the risk of postoperative infection are listed in Table 1–7. In elective cases, many of these factors can be managed preoperatively: Malnutrition or anemia can be corrected, diabetes can be stabilized and, where possible, administration of corticosteroids or other immunosuppressive drugs can be eliminated or decreased to a minimum. Appropriate preoperative evaluation should detect active infection, and adequate treatment can then begin.

Surgical factors that increase the risk of infection are listed in Table 1–8. We have previously discussed the role of different types of surgery with regard to the risk of infection. Interestingly, nighttime and emergency surgery significantly increase the risk. It is most

Table 1–7 Host Factors That Increase the Risk of Wound Infections

Factor	Approximate Increase
Age > 60 years	3x
Malnutrition	3x
Active infection	2-3x
Obesity	2x
Steroid therapy	2x
Diabetes mellitus	2x

Table 1–8. Surgical Factors That Increase the Risk of Wound Infections

Factor	Approximate Increase
Type of wound	
Contaminated	2x
Dirty	4-6x
Preoperative hospitalization	
2 weeks	4x
1-2 weeks	4x
Nighttime or emergency operation	3-4x
Duration of surgery > 3 hours	3-4x
Shaving operation site	2x
Electrosurgical knife	2x
Penrose drain through the wound	2x

important to recognize that the use of the electrosurgical knife also contributes substantially to the risk of postoperative wound infection. It should be noted too that routine use of Penrose drains in clean cases will also significantly increase the rate of postoperative wound infections. In addition, the presence of any foreign body hampers wound healing and adds to the risk of postoperative infection. It has been experimentally demonstrated that even a single suture in the wound can cause infection with a bacterial inoculum that by itself would not result in infection.[59]

In operations with clean-contaminated wounds, there is planned entry into the gastrointestinal tract, the respiratory tract, or the genitourinary tract, all of which have abundant resident microfloras. Even minor spillage is difficult to avoid, despite the most scrupulous surgical technique. It is in this category of clean-contaminated surgery that the greatest need for antimicrobial prophylaxis exists. There are two available approaches to the use of antimicrobial agents in clean-contaminated cases. In the first approach, antibiotics can be used before surgery to decrease the resident flora to such a low level that host defenses can handle the organisms involved in minor spillage without the occurrence of clinically obvious infection. A second approach is to have an antibiotic concentration present in tissues at the time of surgery that is sufficient to kill organisms gaining entry to normally sterile sites.

In contaminated and dirty operations, microorganisms are already present in ordinary sterile sites, and the use of antimicrobial agents represents early therapy rather than prophylaxis. Indeed, antibiotics are mandatory adjuncts in this situation.

Severe malnutrition has adverse effects on wound healing in surgical patients. It is well recognized that extensive surgical procedures in such patients are associated with significant morbidity and mortality. As a result, the use of parenteral hyperalimentation has been recommended to prevent septic and wound complications. Although the use of hyperalimentation is well supported in the management of intestinal fistula and inflammatory intestinal disease, and after massive resection of the small intestine, its short-term value in preventing complications in malnourished patients undergoing surgical procedures is much more controversial.

The role of wound irrigation in preventing wound infection has been debated extensively. In clinical trials, Taylor[60] showed that saline wound irrigation was ineffective in removing bacteria unless the wound was heavily contaminated. This investigator concluded that the only benefit from saline irrigation was the removal of fat or blood clots that could serve as a nidus for infection. Scherr and Dodd[61] reported that a povidone-iodine preparation sterilized aerobic bacteria after a 15-second exposure. Sindelar and Mason[62] reported a significant reduction in infections in potentially contaminated wounds. However, all of their patients were given clindamycin and gentamicin before and after operation. Recently, Galle and Homesley[63] reported that wound infection rates and morbidity were not significantly reduced by the use of povidone-iodine irrigation before closure of the incision in patients not receiving prophylactic antibiotics. However, the weight and volume of evidence suggest that topical antimicrobial therapy is generally helpful in many surgical procedures, with or without systemic administration of drugs.[64,65] Properly, one should choose agents unlikely to be principal systemic drugs of choice to minimize the effect of emerging resistant bacteria. The disadvantages of local antibiotic use are primarily related to the absorption of aminoglycosides, for example, neomycin, with its potentiation of anesthetic ganglionic-blockade.

Intraperitoneal irrigation with solutions containing antibiotics is also controversial.[66] One clinical practice is to irrigate the abdominal cavity in contaminated or potentially contaminated cases with such a solution, usually an aminoglycoside. The efficacy of this technique is not well documented, and where efficacy was demonstrated the authors suggested that the effect was secondary to systemic absorption of the antibiotic from the peritoneal cavity and delivery to local as well as remote tissue sites.[65] Persuasive although unrandomized trials[67,68] in patients with severe established peritonitis suggest particular benefit from a 3-day postoperative regimen of lavage, 1 liter an hour, with the irrigant containing small concentrations of polyantibiotic material. These measures are not justified for true prophylaxis, but may prove of value in severe cases of peritonitis.

The routine use of drains is also controversial. When infection was more common than it is now, drains were often used. However, in their prospective wound surveillance study, Cruse and Foord[58] concluded that drains should not be placed in the operative wound if the wound is to heal without infection. They reported that drains brought through the wound significantly increased the risk of infection.

The best type of drain is a closed suction system, brought out at a distance from the wound. In addition, because infection rates have decreased and surgical skill and techniques have improved, drains are needed less often to drain hematomas or unseen leaks in anastomoses. Smaller suture material leads to less foreign body remaining in wounds, and a need for drains decreases. At present, the only true need for drains is to allow egress of pus and bacteria from established infections or to remove collections of blood or other fluid. In the latter case, suction drains are almost always preferable to simple Penrose drains. When large abscesses are drained, sump pumps are often available, especially if dependent drainage has not been established. Soft sumps are preferable, because the harder drains may cause erosion of bowel and fistula.[69] Routine draining of potential spaces is no longer appropriate.

Although the historic contribution of asepsis has been immense, advances in this area are becoming increasingly expensive and results increasingly difficult to detect. Often the money invested in elaborate operating room designs is far out of proportion to any realistic expectation or results, and some believe that practitioners have reached the maximum that aseptic techniques can offer. Whether this opinion applies to certain refined-clean procedures involving prosthetic implants remains questionable.[70] These techniques will not reduce endogenous flora or contamination already acquired in traumatic wounds. Hunt et al.[71] have suggested that the oldest concept in infection control, that of supporting resistance, is the most fertile source of progress in preventing postoperative infection. The host's susceptibility to infection is universally proportional to the blood supply.

The blood-borne elements of host resistance include leukocytes, complement, interferon, and antibodies. Of the leukocytes, the polymorphonuclear cells are the primary line of defense in acute surgical wounds. When the blood supply is seriously impaired, deprivation of these elements may decrease the ability to resist infection.

It is important to recognize that polymorphonuclear cells need a favorable environment. White cells contain an antibacterial system, the "oxidative pathway." Ingestion of a bacterium excites an oxidative enzyme, which processes dissolved oxygen found in the environment into a family of high-energy oxygen radicals, each of which is toxic to a spectrum of bacteria. These compounds include superoxide, singlet oxygen, hydrogen peroxide, hypochlorite, hypoiodite, and active aldehydes.

The hypoxic white blood cell loses its ability to make these substances. Human cells begin to lose the oxidative pathway at a PO_2 of about 30 mm Hg, which is the range of oxygen tension found in most incised wounds. By the time zero PO_2 is reached, the white blood cell has lost half of its capacity to kill most common wound pathogens. Hunt et al.[71] demonstrated that white blood cells can lose their ability to kill organisms in vivo and that this functional deficiency could be counteracted by supplying more oxygen. To elevate wound oxygen tensions requires a good volume of circulating blood, good cardiac output, and an elevated arterial PO_2. Clinical attempts to elevate wound oxygen supply may be helpful in selected situations.

Although the neutrophil is a primary effector of host defenses, there is much evidence that its function is significantly subnormal in rare instances.[72] Many groups[73] are examining the opsonic process and serum factors as abnormalities much more likely to increase susceptibility to infection.

An additional measure to decrease the risk of postoperative wound infection is to delay primary wound closure in contaminated or dirty cases or in impaired hosts. At surgery the fascia is closed with permanent suture; the subcutaneous space and skin are packed and left open. If the wound appears clean on the fourth postoperative day, the wound is closed. This approach will significantly reduce the risk of infection and does not prolong a hospital stay; the wound heals nearly like a primary closure. The delayed closure is possible because fibroblasts and collagen are not present until the fourth postoperative day, and thus wound healing does not commence until then. Stone and Hester[74] have shown that Neosporin sprayed at the wound edges and primary suture is as efficacious in certain patients as delayed primary closure.

REFERENCES

1. JENSEN NK, JOHNSRUD LW, NELSON MC: Local implantation of sulfanilamide in compound fractures. Surgery 1939;6:1.
2. MELENEY FL: A statistical analysis of a study of the prevention of infection in soft part wounds, compound fractures, and burns with special reference to the sulfonamides. Surg Gynecol Obstet 1945;80:263.
3. BLAKE FG, CRAIGE B Jr, TIERNEY NA: Clinical experiences with penicillin. Trans Assoc Am Physicians 1944;58:67.
4. TUPPER WRC, DAVIS MM: The prophylactic use of penicillin in obstetrics. Am J Obstet Gynecol 1949;57:569.
5. KEETTEL WC, SCOTT JW, PLASS ED: An evaluation of prophylactic penicillin administration to parturient women. Am J Obstet Gynecol 1949;58:335.
6. KEETTEL WC, PLASS ED: Prophylactic administration of penicillin to obstetric patients. JAMA 1950;142:324.
7. SIDDALL RS: Prophylactic penicillin during labor in infection-prone patients. Am J Obstet Gynecol 1950;60:1281.
8. HESSELTINE HC, KEPHART SB: Prophylactic use of penicillin and streptomycin in certain obstetric conditions. Am J Obstet Gynecol 1950;59:184.
9. GUILBEAU JA Jr, SCHOENBACH EB, SCHAUB IG et al: Aureomycin in obstetrics: Therapy and prophylaxis. JAMA 1950;143:520.
10. PRINCE CL: The prevention of urinary tract infection following transurethral prostatic resection by combined use of sulfadiazine and penicillin. J Urol 1946;56:121.
11. GRIFFIN WD, SILVERSTEIN J, HARDT HG Jr et al: Prophylactic chemotherapy in appendicitis. JAMA 1947;133:907.
12. STAFFORD ES: The value of sulfathiazole in the treatment of peritonitis and abscesses of appendical origin. Surg Gynecol Obstet 1942;74:368.
13. PALMER WL, RICKETTS WE: Chronic ulcerative colitis with generalized peritonitis and recovery: Treatment with penicillin and sulfadiazine. Arch Surg 1945;51:102.
14. FAULEY GB, DUGGAN TL, STORMONT RT et al: The use of penicillin in the treatment of peritonitis. JAMA 1944;126:1132.
15. CRILE G Jr, FULTON JR: Appendicitis, with emphasis on the use of penicillin. US Nav Med Bull 1945;45:464.
16. BOWER JO, BURNS JC, MENGLE HA: Prontosil and the treatment of spreading peritonitis in dogs. J Lab Clin Med 1938;24:240.

17. McKITTRICK LS, WHEELOCK FC Jr: The routine use of antibiotics in elective abdominal surgery. Surg Gynecol Obstet 1954; 99:376.

18. MILES AA, MILES EM, BURKE J: The value and duration of defense reactions of the skin to primary lodgment of bacteria. Br J Exp Pathol 1957;38:79.

19. TACHDJIAN MO, COMPERE EL: Postoperative wound infections in orthopedic surgery: Evaluation of prophylactic antibiotics. J Int Coll Surg 1957;28:797.

20. ALLING CC, PULASKI EJ: Current trends in antibiotics in oral surgery. Oral Surg 1959;12:743.

21. SCHRAMEL RJ, CREECH O Jr: Effects of infection and exposure on synthetic arterial prostheses. Arch Surg 1959;78:271.

22. FINLAND M, DAVIDSON CS, LEVENSON SS: Chemotherapy and control of infection among victims of the Cocoanut Grove disaster. Surg Gynecol Obstet 1946;82:151.

23. LYONS C: Problems of infection and chemotherapy. Ann Surg 1943;117:894.

24. LOWBURY EJL: Infection of burns. Br Med J 1960;1:994.

25. TAYLOR GW: Preventive use of antibiotics in surgery. Br Med Bull 1960;16:51.

26. CASON JS, LOWBURY EJL: Prophylactic chemotherapy for burns: Studies on the local and systemic use of combined therapy. Lancet 1960;2:501.

27. ALTEMEIER WA, MacMILLAN BG, HILL EO: The rationale of specific antibiotic therapy in the management of major burns. Surgery 1962;52:240.

28. KEFALIDES NA, ARANA JA, BAZAN A et al: Evaluation of antibiotic prophylaxis and gamma-globulin, plasma, albumin and saline-solution therapy in severe burns: Bacteriologic and immunologic studies. Ann Surg 1964;159:496.

29. WEINSTEIN L: The spontaneous occurrence of new bacterial infections during the course of treatment with strep-tomycin or penicillin. Am J Med Sci 1947;214:56.

30. SMITH DT: The disturbance of the normal bacterial ecology by the administration of antibiotics with the development of new clinical syndromes. Ann Intern Med 1952;37:1135.

31. WEINSTEIN L, GOLDFIELD M, CHANG T-W: Infections occurring during chemotherapy: A study of their frequency, type and predisposing factors. N Engl J Med 1954;251:247.

32. WOODS JW, MANNING IH Jr, PATTERSON CN: Monilial infections complicating the therapeutic use of antibiotics. JAMA 1951;145:207.

33. KEEFER CS: Alterations in normal bacterial flora of man and secondary infections during antibiotic therapy. Am J Med 1951;11:665 (Editorial).

34. POLK HC Jr, STONE HH (eds): Contemporary Burn Management. Boston:Little, Brown, 1971;139–148.

35. MONCRIEF JA, TEPLITZ C: Changing concepts in burn sepsis. J Trauma 1964;4:233.

36. MOYER CA, MARGRAF HW, MONAFO WW Jr: Burn shock and extravascular sodium deficiency: Treatment with Ringer's solution with lactate. Arch Surg 1965;90:799.

37. HAYNES BW Jr: Dextran therapy in severe burns. *In:* Artz CP (ed): Research in Burns. Philadelphia: FA Davis, 1962, p 72.

38. LINDBERG RB, MONCRIEF JA, SWITZER WE et al: The successful control of burn wound sepsis. J Trauma 1965;5:601.

39. POLK HC Jr, MONAFO WW Jr, MOYER CA: Human burn survival: Study of efficacy of 0.5 % aqueous silver nitrate. Arch Surg 1969;98:262.

40. CHODAK GW, PLAUT ME: Use of systemic antibiotics for prophylaxis in surgery. Arch Surg 1977;112:326.

41. DiPIRO JT, RECORD KE, SCHANZENBACH KS et al: Antimicrobial prophylaxis in surgery. I. Am J Hosp Pharm 1981;38:320.

42. SANFORD JP: Prophylactic use of antibiotics: Basic considerations. South Med J 1977;70, Suppl 1:2.

43. VAN SCOY RB: Prophylactic use of antimicrobial agents. Mayo Clin Proc 1977;52:701.

44. GOLDMAN PL, PETERSDORF RG: Prophylactic antibiotics: Controversies give way to guidelines. Drug Ther 1979; June:80.

45. JACOBY I, MANDELL LA, WEINSTEIN L: The chemoprophylaxis of infection: A brief review of recent studies. Med Clin North Am 1978;62:1083.

46. HIRSCHMANN JV, INUI TS: Antimicrobial prophylaxis: A critique of recent trials. Rev Infect Dis 1980;2:1.

47. NEU HC: Clinical pharmacokinetics in preventive antimicrobial therapy. South Med J 1977;70, Suppl 1:14.

48. POLK HC Jr: Prevention of surgical wound infection. Ann Intern Med 1978;89:770.

49. MOELLERING RC Jr, KUNZ LJ, POITRAS JW et al: Microbiologic basis for the rational use of prophylactic antibiotics. South Med J 1977;70, Suppl 1:8.

50. ALLGÖWER M, DÜRIG M, WOLFF G: Infection and trauma. Surg Clin North Am 1980;60:133.

51. POLK HC Jr, LOPEZ-MAYOR JF: Postoperative wound infection: A prospective study of determinant factors and prevention. Surgery 1969;66:97.

52. POLK HC Jr, TRACHTENBERG LS, FINN MP: Antibiotic activity in surgical incisions: The basis of prophylaxis in selected operations. JAMA 1980;244:1353.

53. SHAPIRO M, ALVIRO M, TAGER I, et al: Risk factors for infection at the operative site after abdominal or vaginal hysterectomy. N Engl J Med 1982;307:1661.

54. MacMILLAN BG: Infections following burn injury. Surg Clin North Am 1980;60:185.

55. CUNHA BA, GOSSLING HR, PASTERNAK HS et al: The penetration characteristics of cefazolin, cephalothin, and cephradine into bone in patients undergoing total hip replacement. J Bone Joint Surg 1977;59-A:856.

56. TALLARIDA JR, JACOB LS: The Dose-Response Relation in Pharmacology. New York: Springer, 1981.

57. NATIONAL ACADEMY OF SCIENCE—NATIONAL RESEARCH COUNCIL: Postoperative wound infections: The influence of ultraviolet irradiation of the operating room and of various other factors. Ann Surg 1964;160, Suppl.

58. CRUSE PJE, FOORD R: A five-year prospective study of 23,649 surgical wounds. Arch Surg 1973;107:206.

59. ALEXANDER JW, KAPLAN JZ, ALTEMEIER WA: Role of suture materials in the development of wound infection. Ann Surg 1967;165:192.

60. TAYLOR FW: An experimental evaluation of operative wound irrigation. Surg Gynecol Obstet 1961;113:465.

61. SCHERR DD, DODD TA: In vitro bacteriological evaluation of the effectiveness of antimicrobial irrigating solutions. J Bone Joint Surg 1976;58:119.

62. SINDELAR WF, MASON GR: Efficacy of povidone-iodine irrigation in prevention of surgical wound infection. Surg Forum 1977;28:48.

63. GALLE PC, HOMESLEY HD: Ineffectiveness of povidone-iodine irrigation of abdominal incisions. Obstet Gynecol 1980; 55:744.

64. POLLOCK AV: Topical antibiotics. *In:* Polk HC Jr (ed): Infection and the Surgical Patient. Edinburgh: Churchill Livingstone, 1982;91.

65. POLK HC Jr, FINN MP: Chemoprophylaxis and immunoprophylaxis in surgical wound infection. *In:* Simmons RL,

Howard RJ (eds): Surgical Infectious Disease. New York: Appleton-Century-Crofts, 1982.

66. NOON GP, BEALL AC Jr, DeBAKEY ME: Surgical management of traumatic rupture of the diaphragm. J Trauma 1966; 6:344.

67. STEPHEN M, LOEWENTHAL J: Continuing peritoneal lavage in high-risk peritonitis. Surgery 1979;85:603.

68. RICHARDSON JD, POLK HC Jr: Newer adjunctive treatments for peritonitis. Surgery 1981;90:917.

69. HUBBARD JG, AMIN M, POLK HC Jr: Bladder perforations secondary to surgical drains. J Urol 1979;121:521.

70. POLK HC Jr, GALLAND RB: Infection and host defenses in the surgical patient. *In:* Polk HC Jr (ed): Infection and the Surgical Patient. Edinburgh: Churchill Livingstone; 1982:101.

71. HUNT TK, LINSEY M, GRISLIS H et al: The effect of differing ambient oxygen tensions on wound infection. Ann Surg 1975; 181:35.

72. FUENFER MM, CARR EA Jr, POLK HC Jr: The effect of hydrocortisone on superoxide production by leukocytes. J Surg Res 1979;27:29.

73. KEUSCH GT, DOUGLAS SD, HAMMER G et al: Antibacterial functions of macrophages in experimental protein-calorie malnutrition. II. Cellular and humoral factors for chemotaxis, phagocytosis, and intracellular bactericidal activity. J Infect Dis 1978;138:134.

74. STONE HH, HESTER TR Jr: Incisional and peritoneal infection after emergency celiotomy. Ann Surg 1973;177:669.

Chapter 2

SURGERY OF THE
ALIMENTARY TRACT

Wound and intraabdominal infections remain troublesome sequelae to operations on the alimentary tract. Much can be done to
reduce exogenous contamination of the surgical field by scrupulous
attention to sterile technique.[1] Even the most careful practitioner
encounters situations in which endogenous contamination by intraluminal organisms is unavoidable. This observation is borne out by
the generally high infection rates recorded in different series, and
particularly in colorectal surgery.

Elective operations in which the alimentary tract is opened provide an ideal setting for determination of the effects of antimicrobial
agents on surgical infection rates.[2] The wound is contaminated only
at the time of operation itself; the microbes encountered are more
or less predictable as to genus and species, and the number is
highly variable.

PHARMACOLOGIC CONSIDERATIONS

Chemotherapeutic efforts to modify the host-pathogen encounter
may take four forms:

1. Systemic agents provide circulating antibiotic activity in the
   wound, most especially the incision, when it is made and
   when it is closed, enhancing local tissue resistance but not
   altering the number of microbes spilled.[3]
2. Orally administered, poorly absorbed antibiotics[4] are
   sometimes used in an attempt to lower the intraluminal
   bacterial density and hence reduce the number of bacteria
   delivered to the surgical wound. While this method produces a variable but impressive logarithmic reduction in

27

microbial density, literally millions of bacteria per gram of intestinal contents remain. Some critics of this method allege that the partially absorbed antibiotics do their best work in these regimens by virtue of their systemic absorption.

3. Local or topical application of antimicrobial agents,[5] including antiseptics, depends on direct delivery of antimicrobial activity to the wound edges at time of closure, sacrificing the temporary advantages of preoperative systemic administration but gaining tenfold to twentyfold increases in local activity.

4. Combinations of these methods share complementary rationales. What is curious is that no one has been able to show—in an appropriately randomized study—that combinations of these methods are better than any one method alone. It is hard to imagine that some additive effect does not exist, and it may be the absence of a proper, large, controlled trial that prevents the clinical demonstration of the intellectually obvious.

It is hoped that this organ-oriented review will put much of the available data in perspective and provide a sound rationale and practical basis for selective prophylaxis.

The aim of antibiotic prophylaxis in surgery is to promote adequate bactericidal tissue levels before bacterial contamination of these tissues can take place, thus preventing proliferation of pathogenic organisms in the otherwise more favorable wound environment. Indeed, Polk and Lopez-Mayor[6] originally related the incisional antibiotic activity to the efficacy of prophylaxis. At the same time, prolonged preoperative antibiotic treatment can only encourage the growth of resistant organisms, which may subsequently contaminate the wound. Systemic antibiotic administration should begin just before operation to ensure adequate tissue levels at the time of incision. The use of topical antiseptics and antibiotics for control of incisional infection has been tried in various doses over differing periods of time. These agents, however, are unlikely to influence complications such as bacteremia and intraabdominal abscesses, and their penetration to the depths of the wound is uncertain. Recent reports have called attention to the sometimes dangerously high plasma levels that follow systemic absorption of a locally applied antiseptic or antibiotic. Oral administration may be unsuitable in the immediately preoperative and postoperative periods.

The antibiotic chosen should have high activity against potentially pathogenic organisms normally found in the intestines. Wound infection after gastrointestinal surgery is usually caused by intestinal bacteria, and it is therefore judicious to select a safe drug that is effective against the preponderant bacteria in the large intestine. The antibiotic itself should have few or only mild side effects that do not interfere with anesthesia, hemostasis, or vital organ function. Short-term prophylactic regimens are preferable, although when gross wound contamination occurs, the wound is best considered as already infected and is treated appropriately. In the context of prophylaxis, no benefit appears to accrue from extending the duration of treatment beyond 24 hours. Also, the broadening of the antimicrobial spectrum by adding drugs or substituting those with a wider spectrum has not been shown to provide additional protection.

Antibiotic prophylaxis, particularly in the field of alimentary tract surgery, remains no substitute for careful surgical technique and attention to detail to avoid contamination. In the presence of such considerations, prophylactic antibiotics can have considerable impact on infection rates. The clinical use of systemic antibiotic prophylaxis during the perioperative period for elective gastrointestinal surgery was pioneered by Bernard and Cole.[7] Their patients received penicillin, methicillin, and chloramphenicol before and during surgery and for 5 days afterward. Their infection rate in their patients treated in this manner was 5% compared with 25% in control subjects, but the irregular use of other antibiotics and various stratification problems prevented wide acceptance of their conclusions. Their report, however, did stimulate many subsequent clinical studies of antibiotic prophylaxis.

The use of prophylactic antibiotic therapy in surgery has heretofore been frowned on because the widespread use of antibiotics increases both the development of resistant organisms and the incidence of antibiotic-related complications. Such risks may, however, be diminished by the use of short-term perioperative regimens.

Pseudomembranous colitis is generally regarded as a specific complication of treatment with lincomycin or clindamycin, although there is now some evidence that the penicillins, cephalosporins, and tetracyclines are occasionally implicated as well. The nephrotoxicity or ototoxicity of aminoglycosides precludes their routine use as prophylactic agents.

COLORECTAL SURGERY

Colon aspirates from patients undergoing intestinal surgery yield large numbers of aerobic and anaerobic organisms. *Escherichia coli* is the most common aerobe and *Bacteroides fragilis* the most common anaerobe isolated from postoperative wound infections in gastrointestinal surgery. In addition to these, many kinds of aerobic and anaerobic flora may be involved, usually in mixed culture.

Mechanical preparation of the colon before elective colon surgery is widely practiced, although its value has not been established by randomized trials. Since up to one third of the weight of feces may be bacteria, it appears desirable to remove feces from the operative field in the hope of reducing the threat of infection. However, Nichols et al.[8] showed that although mechanical preparation of the bowel for 3 days before operation effectively removed feces from the colon, the concentration of organisms in the remaining fluid was unchanged.

Prophylactic antibiotic treatment would, therefore, appear to be strongly indicated as an adjunct to mechanical cleansing in the preparation for colonic surgery. To this end, two approaches have been advocated: The first is the oral administration of poorly absorbed antibiotics to reduce the concentration of intestinal bacteria before surgery. The second approach is either oral or parenteral administration of systemically active antibiotics to provide bactericidal wound levels at the time of anticipated contamination.

ORAL PROPHYLAXIS

Poorly absorbed oral antibiotics such as neomycin, kanamycin, and phthalylsulfathiazole, administered for 3 to 5 days before surgery in an attempt to "sterilize" the intestinal lumen, were the subject of several controlled clinical trials during the late 1960s.[9–12] Most of these trials failed to demonstrate any reduction in infection rates with the use of these agents; those that did show some benefit could not achieve infection rates below 30%. Such results bear out the now familiar truism that only an autoclave can sterilize the bowel.

Further trials compared the effectiveness of combinations of poorly absorbed oral antibiotics with that of systemically absorbed oral antibiotics. These studies included neomycin and erythromycin,[8,13] neomycin and tetracycline,[14] neomycin and metronidazole,[15] and kanamycin and metronidazole.[16,17] All of these studies showed highly significant reductions in infection rates to between 5% and 15%. In view of the previous findings with neomycin and kanamycin alone, however, it seems unlikely that the poorly absorbed (intraluminally active) component of such combinations contributes substantially to the observed reductions in infection rates. This is borne out by the findings of Höjer and Wetterfors,[18] who used oral doxycycline alone, and Bjerkeset and Digranes,[19] who used oral metronidazole alone. Each patient in both studies received one preoperative dose, followed by a 5-day postoperative course of antibiotic. Infection rates were reduced from 45% in control groups to 12%[18] and 16%,[19] respectively. As previously noted, however, the use of oral agents in the perioperative period may not be considered desirable in patients undergoing colorectal surgery.

PARENTERAL PROPHYLAXIS

Many controlled studies[6,20–27] were reported in 1969 and the 1970s comparing the effects of parenterally administered prophylactic antibiotics on treated and placebo groups (Table 2–1).

In 7 of these 9 studies, there were highly significant decreases in the incidence of wound infection in antibiotic groups. No further infection rate reductions were apparent in those studies where prophylaxis was continued for 4 or 5 days postoperatively when they were compared with those in which prophylaxis was limited to the day of operation. In the Burton study[21] with gentamicin and the Burdon study[25] with cephalothin, there was no significant change in wound infection rates. Interestingly, in both of these studies no further antibiotic was administered postoperatively.

In the study of Kjellgren and Sellström,[23] cephalothin effectively decreased wound infection, whereas in Burdon's study[25] it did not. A Veterans Administration Cooperative Study,[28] a subsequent multicenter trial, also failed to demonstrate any benefit from the use of cephalothin as a prophylactic antibiotic in colorectal surgery, the overall incidence of complications from infection being 39% in the cephalothin group. Indeed, cephalothin has not been shown to

Table 2-1. Parenteral Systemic Prophylaxis in Colorectal Operations

Author	Antibiotic	Regimen	Infection Rates No. of Patients and % Placebo	Antibiotic	p Value
Polk[6]	Cephaloridine	1 g IM 1 hour preop	15/50 (30%)	4/54 (7%)	= 0.001
Hughes[20]	Penicillin	1 g IM at 5 and 12 hr thereafter 10,000,000 units IV preop	11/44 (25%)	5/50 (10%)	
Burton[21]	Gentamicin	80 mg IM 1 hr preop	12/39 (31%) (wound infection)	14/41 (34%)	
			8/39 (21%) (deep abscess)	4/41 (10%)	
Keighley[22]	Lincomycin	600 mg preop and intraop; then q 8 hr for 5 days	11/29 (38%)	4/23 (17%)	< 0.025
Kjellgren[23]	Cephalothin	2 g preop and intraop; then 2 g q 6 hr for 4 days	26/49 (53%)	10/57 (17%)	< 0.001
Feathers[24]	Lincomycin plus gentamicin	Given for 5 days: 1.6 mg/kg q 8 hr adjusted to maintain serum levels at 3-10 µg/ml for 5 days	12/45 (48%)	0/13 (0%)	
	or				
	Metronidazole	1 g as suppository or IV q 8 hr for 5 days			
	plus gentamicin	1.6 mg/kg q 8 hr adjusted to maintain serum levels at 3-10 µg/ml for 5 days		1/14 (7%)	
Burdon[25]	Cephalothin	1 or 2 g preop and 1 hr later	24/47 (51%)	18/46 (39%)	
Galland[26]	Lincomycin plus tobramycin	600 mg IM preop and at 8 hr 160 mg IM preop and at 8 hr	16/38 (42%)	3/37 (8%)	= 0.02
Eykyn[27]	Metronidazole	500 mg IV preop and at 8 and 16 hr postop	30/39 (77%)	15/44 (34%)	< 0.005

Preop, preoperatively; intraop, intraoperatively; postop, postoperatively; IM, intramuscularly; IV, intravenously.

be a consistently effective agent in alimentary tract procedures. To some degree, this failure of cephalothin prophylaxis may be due to its rapid disappearance from the tissue at the surgical incision site, a characteristic not shared by cefazolin and cephaloridine, the consistently clinically effective cephalosporins.[29] The increasing incidence of wound infections due to cephalosporin-resistant aerobes highlights the problems that may occur when the widespread use of an antibiotic promotes the development of bacterial strains resistant to it.

Gentamicin, which acted poorly in the Burton study, is effective in vitro against coliforms, staphylococci, and *Pseudomonas* species. It appeared to act more effectively in a study by Feathers et al.,[24] in which it was combined with either lincomycin or metronidazole, both of which are effective against anaerobes. Because pseudomembranous colitis developed in 2 of the patients treated with lincomycin, Feathers et al. concluded that lincomycin was unacceptable as a prophylactic agent in colorectal surgery. Overuse of gentamicin increases the number of resistant organisms, and close serum monitoring is required with its use to ensure effective antibiotic levels while preventing toxic accumulation. Nevertheless, in this study no overt problems with gentamicin toxicity were observed; this suggests both the safety and the efficacy of a regimen of gentamicin plus metronidazole to prevent infection in colorectal surgery.

Despite this finding, reservations exist concerning the widespread use of a drug such as gentamicin, an agent associated with identifiable significant complications, as a propylactic agent. The potential exists to do more harm than good to the patient. The trial of Eykyn et al.[27] with metronidazole alone also showed a highly significant reduction in infection rates. The infection rate of 34% in the metronidazole group may reflect risk factors in the patient population, as the rate of infection of their placebo group was unusually high (77%). A study by Bjerkeset and Digranes[19] of orally administered metronidazole showed a reduction in infection rates to 16%, and toxicity with metronidazole does not appear to be as severe a problem as with gentamicin.

Most of these trials dealt with too few subjects to permit conclusions with regard to mortality. A recent review[30] combining data from a number of reports concludes that antibiotic prophylaxis for colorectal surgery does decrease postoperative mortality. Thus, the benefits to the patient undergoing colorectal surgery, in terms of reduced morbidity and mortality, appear to outweigh the disadvantages associated with the use of prophylactic antibiotics, such as the development of resistant strains and potential toxicity. Such disadvantages may be offset by the judicious choice of antibiotic and by using it for the shortest effective period of time.

APPENDECTOMY

The use of prophylactic antibiotics in acute appendicitis has been widely studied. Although infection rates in nonperforated appendicitis may be as low as 6%,[31] they may be as high as 90% if the appendix is perforated.[32] Prophylactic antibiotics can, therefore, be expected to have a considerable impact on morbidity, especially in patients with perforated appendices; controlled trials have borne this out.

Microbiology

Leigh et al.[33] cultured specimens from the appendix fossa in 322 patients undergoing appendectomy. Bacteria were recovered from 49% of their patients, the most common organisms being *Bacteroides* sp. (74%), *Klebsiella/Enterobacteriaceae* sp. (29%), and *E. coli* (25%). Their overall wound infection rate was 19%, the most common isolate being *Bacteroides* sp.; these were also found in the appendix fossa cultures. Although anaerobic organisms appear to predominate, it is interesting to note that the reductions in infection rates achieved with antibiotics effective against aerobic organisms were similar to those effective against anaerobes. This latter finding is not unique to appendectomy. Curiously, the aerobe-specific or anaerobe-specific therapy produces similar overall control rates; according to limited published data, they do not appear to be additive when used in combination.

Clinical Studies

Several controlled trials[31,32,34–43] using either topical or systemic antibiotic prophylaxis in acute appendicitis are summarized in

Table 2–2. Significant decreases in wound infection were associated with topical ampicillin, topical polyantibiotic spray or povidone-iodine spray, rectal and parenteral metronidazole, ornidazole, clindamycin, or cephaloridine. Single-dose cefazolin, however, failed to show any beneficial effect. Infection rates with antibiotic prophylaxis varied from 0.5% to 5.8% in patients with nonperforated appendices, and from 7% to 31% in patients with perforation in those series in which a beneficial effect was demonstrated.

A further study by Fine and Busuttil[44] attempted to correlate the antimicrobial spectrum with the anticipated pathogens. They used a combination of clindamycin and gentamicin, and reduced the sepsis rate from 10.2% in nonperforated appendicitis to 5.3% in the prophylaxis group. As noted in the previous section, however, neither antibiotic is without risk of significant complications; this finding raises questions as to the wisdom of their use as prophylactic agents in appendicitis.

More recently, attempts have been made to rationalize prophylactic antibiotic treatment in appendicitis by differentiating between perforated and nonperforated cases. Gottrup,[42] in a study of more than 400 patients, compared placebo with metronidazole, streptomycin, and penicillin. Before operation all patients received either placebo or 500 mg intravenous metronidazole. Patients with nonperforated appendices received no further treatment. Patients with gangrenous or perforated appendices received topical penicillin and streptomycin and, postoperatively, systemic metronidazole, streptomycin, and penicillin for 5 days. In the nonperforated group, infection rates were reduced from 3.7% (5/135) to 0.75% (1/133). In the gangrenous/perforated group, infection rates were reduced from 53% (23/43) to 0 (0/66). The author noted that, in the bacteriologic data, the use of penicillin was redundant, but suggested that a suitable rationale would be to give all patients with acute appendicitis a single preoperative dose of metronidazole. Those with normal or acutely inflamed appendices do not require any further antibiotic. If the appendix is gangrenous or perforated, treatment is continued with metronidazole plus a suitable antibiotic effective against aerobic organisms.

Most of these studies demonstrate the considerable impact that prophylactic antibiotics can have on postoperative morbidity due to infection in acute appendicitis. Moreover, several different antibiotics have been shown to be effective, in some instances even after a single preoperative dose.

Table 2-2. Appendectomy and Antibiotic Prophylaxis (Topical or Systemic, or Both)

| Author | Antibiotic | Regimen | Infection Rates No. of Patients and % | | |
			Placebo	Antibiotic	p Value
Palmu[31]	Ornidazole	750 mg IV immediately preop:			
		(a) nonperforated appendices	5/89 (6%)	5/86 (6%)	
		(b) perforated appendices	7/11 (64%)	1/14 (17%)	
Andersen[32]	Topical ampicillin	1 g sprinkled into wound before closing:			
		(a) nonperforated appendices	16/187 (9%)	1/187 (1%)	< 0.01
		(b) perforated appendices	26/29 (90%)	9/29 (31%)	
Rickett[34]	Topical ampicillin	500 mg sprinkled into wound before closing. 15% of patients given unspecified postop antibiotics	16/66 (24%)	2/64 (3%)	< 0.01
Gilmore[35]	Polyantibiotic spray	Neomycin-bacitracin-polymyxin powder spray into wound before closing	15/84 (18%)	8/84 (10%)	< 0.04
	Povidone-iodine spray	Before closing		7/84 (8%)	

Reference	Antibiotic	Regimen			p
Bates[36]	Topical ampicillin	500 mg into wound before closing	16/100 (16%)	3/100 (3%)	< 0.01
Willis[37]	Metronidazole	1 g suppository preop. Then q 8 hr postop until oral feeding, then 200 mg per os q 8 hr until day 7	14/46 (30%)	2/49 (4%)	< 0.05
Everson[38]	Cephaloridine	1 g q 6 hr for 3 days	34/126 (27%)	14/120 (12%)	
Foster[39]	Cephaloridine	12.5 mg/kg q 6 hr for 2 days	8/69 (12%)	1/70 (1%)	< 0.02
Greenall[40]	Metronidazole	500 mg IV immediately preop	12/51 (24%)	1/49 (2%)	= 0.02
Donovan[41]	Clindamycin	600 mg IV in OR	24/72 (33%)	14/81 (17%)	< 0.05
	Cefazolin	1 g IV in OR		30/85 (35%)	
Gottrup[42]	Metronidazole	500 mg IV in OR. Perforated appendices: metronidazole, penicillin and streptomycin postop (see text)	28/206 (14%)	1/200 (1%)	< 0.001
Bates[43]	Metronidazole	500 mg into wound before closing	21/83 (25%)	17/87 (20%)	

Postop, postoperatively; preop, preoperatively; OR, operating room; IV, intravenously.

GASTRODUODENAL SURGERY

Microbiology

Gray and Shiner[45] and Drasar et al.[46] showed that there are no or few microorganisms in the normal human stomach. However, the stomachs of patients with gastric ulcer or gastric cancer contain larger numbers of bacteria than those of patients with duodenal ulcer or normal stomachs. Gatehouse et al.[47] reported that the rate of wound infection associated with gastric surgery correlated with preoperative bacterial counts obtained by gastric aspiration. Thus, wound infection rates, without antibiotic prophylaxis, were 17%, 38%, and 56% after surgery for duodenal ulcer, gastric ulcer, and gastric carcinoma, respectively. The preponderant organisms recovered were aerobes, and frequently were those found in the nasopharyngeal flora (Table 2–3).

Moreover, these investigators[47] showed that wound infection was caused by one or more organisms found in the gastric aspirate, especially when total viable counts exceeded 5×10^6 organisms/ml. Thus, the wound infection rate was higher in patients operated on for gastric cancer (56%) than for duodenal ulcer (17%). The authors suggested that antibiotic prophylaxis may not be indicated for all patients undergoing gastric surgery. Clinical signs, possibly supplemented by preoperative quantitative gastric cultures, can identify those patients at the highest risk.

Table 2–3. Organisms Isolated From the Stomach and Wound Infections After Gastric Surgery

Lactobacilli	Haemophilus sp.
Streptococcus viridans*	Staphylococcus albus*
Yeasts	Bifidobacteria
Micrococci	Proteus sp.*
Streptococcus faecalis*	Nonhemolytic streptococci
Diphtheroids	Staphylococcus aureus*
Escherichia coli*	Klebsiella aerogenes
Neisseria sp.	Anaerobic streptococci*
Clostridium sp.*	Veillonella sp.
Bacteroides sp.*	β-Hemolytic streptococci*

*Organism subsequently isolated from wound infections.
Adapted from Gatehouse et al.,[47] with permission.

Clinical Studies

Table 2–4 summarizes 10 reports in the English-language literature dealing with the use of antibiotic prophylaxis in gastroduodenal surgery. Earlier authors[48–50] were unable to report a beneficial effect of prophylaxis. These studies were not randomized; the investigators used multiple antibiotic regimens, and prophylaxis was initiated postoperatively or its time of initiation was not specified.

In the randomized studies in which prophylaxis was initiated preoperatively, wound infection rates varied from 22% to 63% in the control groups compared with 0 to 5% in the prophylaxis groups.[6,51–56] In each of these studies perioperative prophylaxis significantly reduced postoperative wound infection associated with gastric surgery. A combination of penicillin, methicillin, and chloramphenicol[51] was effective, as were cefazolin[54,56] and cephaloridine.[6,55] To date there is no evidence that newer cephalosporins provide more protection as prophylactic agents.[57] Single-dose intraoperative prophylaxis with lincomycin and tobramycin reduced wound infection rates from 34% to 5%.[53]

Pories et al.[56] studied the value of cefazolin prophylaxis in gastric bypass surgery for obesity. In 53 patients, the wound infection rate was reduced from 21% to 4%. These authors also found that urinary and respiratory tract infections were reduced in this high-risk group of patients from 17% to 0 ($p < 0.05$), an observation not usually reported in other trials of attempted perioperative systemic prophylaxis.

Lewis[55] confirmed the bacteriologic observations of Gatehouse et al.[47] in a prospective clinical study. Patients were randomly assigned to the following risk and prophylaxis groups:

Group I   Low risk: no antibiotics
Group II High risk: perioperative cephaloridine (surgery for duodenal ulcer complicated by pyloric stenosis, or for peptic or gastric ulcer or malignancy)
Group III High-risk controls: no antibiotic

No wound infections occurred in the low-risk patients (group I). Eleven of the 42 (26%) group III patients (high-risk, without prophylaxis) had subsequent wound infections, but none of the 41 group II patients (high-risk, with prophylaxis) had such infections. The incidence of respiratory and urinary tract infections was not

Table 2-4. Published Reports on Prophylactic Antibiotics in Gastroduodenal Surgery

Author	Study Randomized (R) or Not (NR)	Timing of Antibiotics	No Antibiotics Given		Antibiotics		p Value
			No. of Patients	Wound Infection	No. of Patients	Wound Infection	
Polk[6]	R	Perioperative	36	11 (31%)	32	0	< 0.001
McKittrick[48]	NR	Not stated	24	0	36	1 (3%)	NS
Barnes[49]	NR	Postoperative	1,212	94 (8%)	1,459	89 (6%)	NS
Sonneland[50]	NR	Postoperative	85	5 (6%)	104	12 (12%)	NS
Feltis[51]	R	Perioperative	64	14 (22%)	40	2 (5%)	< 0.02
Evans[52]	R	Perioperative	30	6 (20%)	33	1 (3%)	< 0.05
Griffiths[53]	R	Preoperative	8	5 (62%)	5	0	< 0.05
Stone[54]	R	Perioperative	23	5 (22%)	49	0	< 0.02
Lewis[55]	R	Perioperative	42	11 (26%)	41	0	< 0.02
Pories[56]	R	Perioperative	23	5 (22%)	27	1 (4%)	< 0.05

NS, not significant.

significantly different in the three groups; this finding is in contrast to the observations of Pories et al.[56] Lewis[55] noted that cimetidine, a histamine H_2-receptor antagonist, may be responsible for the reduced numbers in the low-risk group.

The evidence shows that perioperative prophylaxis reduces the rate of wound infection after gastric surgery. The wound infection rate is ordinarily low after elective surgery for duodenal ulcer and therefore antibiotic prophylaxis is not usually warranted. Those patients with impairment of mechanisms (gastric motility and acidity) that normally restrict the growth of organisms are at higher risk of infection. Thus, patients with achlorhydria or gastric ulcer or malignancy should receive perioperative prophylaxis.

HEPATOBILIARY SURGERY

Microbiology

The bacteriology of the biliary tract has been investigated by many authors.[58-62] The normal gallbladder and bile are either sterile or yield small numbers of microorganisms.[58,59] Bile cultures are positive in 10% to 100% of patients with chronic cholecystitis, choledocholithiasis, or postoperative biliary constriction.[59-65] Over a 5-year period, bile cultures were positive in 33% of the 1,421 biliary operations. Chetlin and Elliott[62] described valid clinical signs that correlate with a genuine high-risk state among patients undergoing operation for biliary tract disease.

The organisms found in infected bile are gram-negative rods, most commonly *E. coli,* and *Streptococcus faecalis.* Certain less common organisms, such as lactobacilli, microaerophilic streptococci, *Bacillus* sp., *Streptococcus viridans* and staphylococci have also been recovered.[66-70] Anaerobes, including *Clostridium* sp., are sometimes present, but these organisms do not appear to be important causes of postoperative infection; indeed, metronidazole prophylaxis has been demonstrated to be of no value in biliary tract surgery.[66]

Since the incidence of postoperative wound infection is higher in patients with positive bile cultures, attempts have been made to correlate "risk factors" with "bactibilia" and the rate of postoperative wound infection.[64] Other authors have attempted to use intraoperative Gram stains of bile as a guide to prophylaxis[71] or the quantitation of bacteria found in preoperative duodenal aspirates.[72] Neither of these two techniques has gained widespread acceptance.

By using multivariate analysis, Keighley and Alexander-Williams[64] identified eight "high-risk factors" that preoperatively predict the likelihood of positive bile cultures (Table 2–5); these factors are extensions of Chetlin and Elliott's[62] original proposals.

The incidence of positive biliary cultures, wound infections, and bacteremia after surgery was higher in 45 "high-risk" patients than in 136 "low-risk" patients.

E. coli, Klebsiella sp. and *Proteus* sp. are the gram-negative organisms most commonly found in postoperative wound infections associated with biliary tract surgery.[52,71] *Staphylococcus aureus* is the most common gram-positive organism and, in some series, the most common cause of postoperative biliary tract wound infection.[52,71,73] *S. faecalis* is far more commonly isolated from infected bile than *S. aureus*, but its role as a surgical pathogen is still debatable. This finding suggests that organisms found in the bile or on the patient's skin, or acquired in the operating room can all be responsible for postoperative infection. The antibiotic used for prophylaxis, therefore, must be active against staphylococci and Enterobacteriaceae, particularly *E. coli, Klebsiella* sp. and *Proteus* sp.; *S. faecalis* and anaerobes are less important.

Pharmacology and Clinical Studies

The choice of antibiotic for prophylaxis should take into account the drug's in vivo activity against the presumed pathogens. The drug theoretically should be able to penetrate the target tissues, for

Table 2–5. High-Risk Infection Factors in Operations on the Biliary Tract

---
Age over 70 years
Jaundice at operation
Stress within 1 week of operation
Emergency operation
Operation within 4 weeks before emergency admission
Previous biliary operation
Stones in the bile duct
Bile duct obstruction

Adapted from Keighley and Alexander-Williams,[64] with permission.

example, the wound or gallbladder wall, in adequate concentrations for the duration of the operation. Cephalosporins seem a logical choice in biliary tract surgery because they are active against *S. aureus* and most enteric bacteria. Ampicillin has less activity against these organisms but is indicated when enterococci are the presumed pathogen. Gentamicin is more consistently active against the usual enteric bacteria than are the older cephalosporins; in addition, it is active in vitro against staphylococci and thus is a theoretic alternative to the cephalosporins for the prophylaxis of patients undergoing cholecystectomy.

Cunha et al.[74] found that among 2,902 cholecystectomy patients, 25 had wound infections after surgery. Of 1,735 patients who did not receive prophylactic antibiotics, 24 (1.4%) had wound infections, whereas, of the 1,167 patients who were given such therapy, only 1 had a wound infection. All antibiotics were given by intravenous bolus injection immediately before operation. In the prophylaxis group, cefazolin (94%) was the most commonly used cephalosporin (72%), ampicillin was used in 24% of the patients, and gentamicin was used in the remaining 4%. The single *S. aureus* wound infection in the prophylaxis group was in a patient who received ampicillin. Although cephalosporins are, in general, less effective against gram-negative organisms than aminoglycosides, there was no wound infection in any patient receiving cephalosporin prophylaxis. Gentamicin appeared to be a reasonable alternative to the cephalosporins for biliary tract prophylaxis since both *S. aureus* and *E. coli* were inhibited by this antibiotic. These investigators concluded that a single parenteral preoperative dose of an antibiotic was the best regimen for preventing wound infections associated with cholecystectomy. The prophylaxis need not be continued for more than 24 hours after surgery since wound infections originate during the operation.

The current trend has, in fact, been to reduce the duration of prophylaxis. Strachan et al.[67] compared the incidence of wound infections after elective biliary surgery in control subjects, patients receiving a single dose, and patients having a 5-day course of cefazolin; this study too demonstrated the efficacy of single-dose prophylaxis. Although the antibiotic did not affect the rate of organisms from the bile at surgery, the single-dose regimen caused a significant reduction in the rate of wound infections from 11 of 65 (17%) in the control group to 2 of 63 (3%) in the antibiotic group. Four of 73 patients (5.5%) having the 5-day course subsequently had wound infections; this percentage was not significantly different from that of the control group. Wound infections were significantly more frequent when the bile was infected at the time of surgery and when the common duct was explored. The average hospital stay was significantly longer among patients with wound infections than among those without wound infections. Intraperitoneal infection did not develop in any patient in any group.

The administration of prophylactic antibiotics before surgery, so that adequate tissue levels can be achieved at the time of contamination, also appears to be important. Strachan et al.,[67] in a trial with patients undergoing biliary surgery, showed that preoperative administration of cefazolin reduced the rate of wound infection to 2%. When prophylaxis was begun after the operation, the infection rate was similar to that in the control group.

It is difficult to determine from these studies how useful antimicrobial prophylaxis is for *all* cases of elective biliary tract surgery. High-risk patients require protection; healthy young people undergoing cholecystectomy when common-duct exploration is unnecessary do not require protection. Since the need for choledochoscopy cannot be predicted with more than 85% accuracy, a rational plan might well be to administer a single preoperative dose of a proven, wound-active agent. If the common duct is opened, then two or three additional doses should be administered.

ABDOMINAL TRAUMA

Penetrating abdominal injuries and blunt abdominal trauma with intestinal perforation are considered contaminated wounds (class IV; see Appendix, Guideline) requiring antibiotic therapy. Although this is anticipatory therapy, the principles are sufficiently similar to warrant discussion here. Studies of the use of systemic antibiotics in these situations correctly do not include placebo groups.

Microbiology

Aerobic infection is common after surgery for abdominal trauma. *E. coli* was the most common and *S. aureus* the second most common organism isolated from the wound and the peritoneal cavity in 102 trauma patients reported by Matolo et al.[75] The importance of anaerobic bacteria in abdominal trauma has been emphasized by Thadepalli et al.[76] In their study, 100 patients with abdominal trauma and surgical exploration received either cephalothin and kanamycin or clindamycin and kanamycin. In 9 of 52 patients receiving cephalothin and kanamycin, anaerobic infections developed in 6 patients postoperatively, necessitating a change of therapy. Infection necessitated a change of therapy in 3 of 48 patients receiving clindamycin and kanamycin, but only one of these infections was due to an anaerobic organism (*Clostridium* sp.). Thadepalli et al. predictably concluded that anaerobes are a significant cause of infection in patients with abdominal trauma and that clindamycin and kanamycin should be used in these situations.

Pharmacology and Clinical Studies

Topical therapy has also been studied in abdominal trauma. In one study[77] of topical kanamycin therapy, the wound infection rate was 10% (12/124 patients) in the kanamycin group and 20% (23/116 patients) in the placebo group. Of 240 patients entered into the study, 57 also received systemic prophylaxis or treatment for various indications in nonrandomized fashion. Thus, of the remaining 183 patients who received no systemic antibiotics, 96 received placebo topical therapy and 87 received topical kanamycin therapy. The wound infection rate in the former group was 19% and in the latter 7% ($p = 0.05$). The authors concluded that topical kanamycin was of value in reducing wound infection rates after abdominal trauma. In addition, a high infection rate was confirmed in patients receiving neither parenteral nor topical antibiotic prophylaxis.

Fullen et al.[78] retrospectively studied 295 patients with penetrating abdominal trauma. Patients were divided into three groups: Group A had preoperative and postoperative antibiotic prophylaxis, group B had intraoperative and postoperative prophylaxis, and group C received only postoperative antibiotic prophylaxis. The antibiotic regimens, which were not standardized, consisted of unspecified combinations of penicillin, chloramphenicol, and tetracycline. The total infection rate was significantly reduced in group A (7%) when compared with those of group B (33%) and group C (30%).

The rates of deep infection and wound infection in the three groups are summarized in Figure 2–1. Mortality in each group was

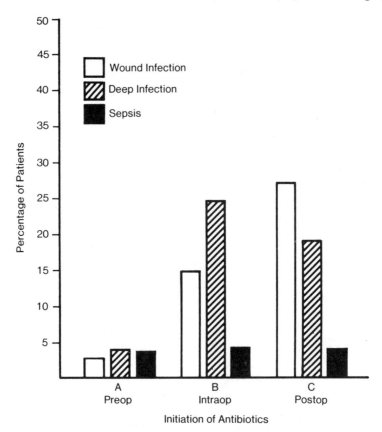

Fig. 2–1. Distribution of infection rates (wound infection, deep infection or septicemia) in groups treated initially before (preop), during (intraop) and after (postop) operation. From Fullen et al.,[78] with permission.

4%. Fullen et al. concluded that preoperative and intraoperative antibiotic administration offers a significant advantage when compared with intraoperative or postoperative initiation of therapy in the prevention of posttraumatic wound or deep infection.

Crenshaw et al.[79] studied 200 nonrandomized patients requiring "emergency procedures." Cephalothin and tobramycin were given intravenously preoperatively and postoperatively for 72 hours. The overall infection rate in this series of patients was low (2%); the authors attributed this low rate to the effectiveness of the antibiotic regimen and to painstaking surgical technique.

In a retrospective study of 721 patients undergoing emergency laparotomy, however, Stone and Hester[80] concluded that cephalothin administration, whether given preoperatively and post-operatively or postoperatively alone, failed to prevent wound infection. The incidence of peritoneal abscess was halved (5.6%) when cephalothin was initiated preoperatively rather than post-operatively (12.4%). Firm conclusions cannot be drawn from this study about the use of antibiotics in abdominal trauma because of the use of historical controls and because of the inclusion of patients having emergency surgery for differing reasons, for example, perforated ulcer or appendicitis. The inadequacy of cephalothin as a prophylactic agent has been previously discussed.

In a similar retrospective analysis, which included only patients with penetrating abdominal trauma, O'Donnell et al.[81] concluded that a combination of preoperative clindamycin (600 mg every 6 hours) and gentamicin (80 mg every 6 hours) significantly reduced the intraabdominal infection rate from 8.3% to 1.7% when compared with an "uncontrolled" group, which underwent standard antibiotic regimens. The study, however, is retrospective and non-randomized, and lacks supporting microbiologic data.

In a subsequent report, O'Donnell et al.[82] compared carbenicillin alone with clindamycin and gentamicin. This study was randomized and prospective but not blinded, and included 126 patients undergoing emergency laparotomy for penetrating abdominal trauma. Nine patients were excluded from the analysis because of unfavorable findings at surgery. Of the remaining 117 patients, 5 who were given carbenicillin and 6 who were given clindamycin and gentamicin experienced unspecified "infectious complications." This difference was not significant statistically. The authors concluded that the overall infection rate of 9.4% compared favorably with that reported in the literature; however, concurrent untreated controls were not included in this trial.

In a similar uncontrolled study by Matolo et al.[75] in 1976, intraoperative clindamycin and gentamicin were administered intravenously to trauma patients with intestinal or biliary perfora-tion. In 102 patients, the wound infection rate was 4%; abdominal abscesses and septicemia occurred in 2.9% and 1%, respectively. The mortality was 3.9% (4/102); however, only one of these was attributed to an infectious complication. The authors concluded that their overall infection rate of 7.9% was lower than that previously reported and that parenteral and intraperitoneal antibiotic use was of value in preventing postoperative infection associated with trauma.

Surgical exploration for abdominal trauma is associated with a high rate of postoperative infection and is classified as contaminated (class IV). Antibiotic use is regarded as therapeutic rather than prophylactic, and is recommended. Aerobic and anaerobic gastrointestinal organisms such as *E. coli* and *B. fragilis*, along with *S. aureus*, are important causes of infectious complications.

DISCUSSION

Antibiotic prophylaxis has a significant impact on infection rates in all types of surgery involving the colon or appendix, and after abdominal trauma. It is effective also in selected patients undergoing hepatobiliary or gastroduodenal surgery. The most beneficial effects are noted when the antibiotic is given before surgery so that tissue levels are adequate at the time of contamination. To discourage the development of resistant bacterial strains, the initial antibiotic dose should be administered parenterally immediately prior to operation; except in grossly contaminated cases, no benefit appears to accrue from prolonging prophylactic treatment beyond 24 hours. The judicious choice of an antibiotic for prophylaxis can help to diminish the potential for drug-related toxicity. The overall benefits of antibiotic prophylaxis are demonstrated by the reduction in infection-related morbidity and mortality achieved in patients undergoing gastrointestinal surgery.

The reviews described provide valuable information about the difficult science of interpreting and utilizing data from large noncomparable trials. Elective operations, the proper forum for true prophylaxis, on certain organs allow the wisest choices. Patients undergoing transabdominal operations, in which the colon or rectum is opened, benefit from perioperative systemic antibiotics and from oral, poorly absorbable antibiotics given before operation. They seem similarly efficacious, but, curiously, no one has shown that these benefits are in any way additive.

Elective gastroduodenal operations require further categorization: If acid production is low or absent, as in patients with gastric ulcer, gastric cancer, or cimetidine-treated duodenal ulcer, intragastric bacteria are much like those in the colon, and systemic prophylaxis is protective and generally warranted. If acid production is normal, for example, in patients with intractable duodenal ulcer, then gastric microbes are sparse or absent, and there is no measurable benefit from prophylaxis.

Elective biliary tract operations similarly require stratification.

Simple cholecystectomy, with or without cholangiography, has a very low infection rate, and prophylaxis is therefore probably not justified. On the other hand, conditions that warrant common bile duct exploration, notably jaundice, advanced age, or subsiding acute cholecystitis, show a high incidence of "bactibilia," and these patients should be treated with systemic antibiotic prophylaxis. Biliary excretion of an agent does not correlate with prophylactic efficacy.

The use of antibiotics for appendectomy and penetrating abdominal trauma for semantic purists represents early therapy, rather than exemplary prophylaxis. Systemic antibiotics upon diagnosis are mandatory if clinical signs suggest perforation—free or localized—or abscess formation (or both). The value of systemic drugs in nonperforative appendicitis remains moot; if doubt exists based on clinical signs, then surely little harm is done by a single preoperative dose of a safe antibiotic, letting operative findings determine whether further treatment is warranted and for how long.

The same principle applies to penetrating abdominal trauma; some 10% to 15% of injuries are not in bacteria-laden organs, but the vast majority of injuries are associated with very real contamination. Therefore, the wisest course is to initiate specific therapy in the *first* bottle of resuscitative fluids and to let operative findings determine the duration of therapy.

If the foregoing queries and answers determine "who" should have prophylaxis, then "when" must be obvious: prior to contamination in elective procedures and as soon as the diagnosis is made in the early therapy situation.

"What" drug to use is a more difficult decision by far. Systemic prophylaxis should be examined first. The weight of evidence in properly conducted trials favors cephaloridine, but the nephrotoxicity of this antibiotic has appropriately limited its current availability in the United States. Cefazolin is the next best studied agent. Therein lies an observation that gnaws at the basis of prophylaxis directed against anaerobic microbes that inhabit the alimentary tract. The shift to the so-called second- and third-generation cephalosporins, with better anti-anaerobic activity, has not improved the typical 7% infection rate that attended trials of the aerobe-specific first-generation drugs.

The specific problem of the frequent use of cephalothin in reported trials distorts much of the data available in these important clinical areas. Cephalothin, unlike cefazolin or cephaloridine, does not reliably lower incisional infection rates, presumably because of its rapid disappearance from surgical wounds. Cephalosporins with longer serum and tissue half-lives may thus prove to be more effective. Further investigation in this area is necessary.

Which oral regimen to use is a much more difficult determination. Again, a number of investigators would favor neomycin plus erythromycin base,[4] although there are disturbing reports of failure in some trials.[83] Treatment should probably be aimed at both aerobic and anaerobic bacteria, although whether slightly absorbable agents are better than the truly nonabsorbable ones is unknown.[84] The most stringent and best controlled study[14] of colorectal surgery found that neomycin/tetracycline was efficacious. To further the confusion, the degree to which the remarkable British experience with metronidazole can be reproduced in North America is largely unknown.[83]

Whichever regimen is chosen, real and potential safety should supersede even efficacy and spectrum. Most patients not treated with antibiotics will have *no* infections. One needs to be certain that the disease prevented is worse—and more frequent—than the complications of the selected method of prophylaxis.

For fear that one may carry the skepticism about the need for complete (that is, aerobe and anaerobe) coverage for prophylaxis too far, the need for therapy in documented examples of anaerobic infection is sound and unquestioned. Indeed, there is a parallel with the inability to demonstrate additive effects of systemic and oral prophylaxis for colorectal operations; some trials of attempted systemic prophylaxis in gynecologic surgery show identical clinical infection rates after either aerobe-specific or anaerobe-specific agents with, again, no additive effects of the pair. It may well be that effective therapy with either of the symbiotic pair produces a clinically similar outcome and that at least in prophylaxis, attacks on both are not further protective.

New agents not yet subject to refereed publication of randomized prospective trials also suffer in these comparisons.

PRACTICAL SURGICAL RECOMMENDATIONS

1. For elective gastroduodenal operations associated with normal gastric acidity and for high-risk biliary tract operations, these regimens are recommended:

    a. Cefazolin, 1 g intramuscularly on call to the operating room and one or two additional doses on the day of operation;
    or

    b. Gentamicin or tobramycin, 1.75 mg/kg of body weight intramuscularly, on call to the operating room and one or two additional doses on the day of operation for biliary tract cases only.

2. For elective colorectal operations, in addition to scrupulous mechanical cleansing, these regimens are recommended:

    a. Cefazolin, 1 g intramuscularly, on call to the operating room and one or two additional doses on the day of operation;
    or

    b. Cefoxitin, 1 g intravenously, on call to the operating room and one or two additional doses on the day of operation;
    or

    b. Neomycin and erythromycin base, 1 g each orally at 1 p.m., 2 p.m. and 11 p.m. on the day before the operation;
    or

    b. Neomycin and tetracycline, 500 mg neomycin and 250 mg tetracycline orally every 6 hours for 48 hours preoperatively;
    or

    c. Metronidazole, 500 mg intravenously, on call to the operating room and at 8 and 16 hours postoperatively.

3. In situations requiring early therapy, the first bottle of resuscitative fluids should contain:

    a. Cefazolin, 2 g, followed by 3 to 4 g/day, depending on body weight and degree of contamination;
    or

    b. Cefoxitin, 2 g, followed by 4 to 6 g/day, depending on body weight and degree of contamination;
    or

    c. Clindamycin, 600 mg, followed by similar amounts every 6 hours, and tobramycin 1.5 mg/kg of body weight every 8 hours intramuscularly or intravenously, depending on the degree of contamination.

REFERENCES

1. FLINT LM, FRY DE (eds): Surgical Infections: Discussions in Surgical Management. Garden City, NY: Medical Examination Publishing Co., 1982.
2. POLK HC Jr, AUSOBSKY JR: The role of antibiotics in surgical infections. *In:* MacLean LD (ed): Advances in Surgery. Chicago: Year Book Medical Publishers; 1983: 225–275.
3. GALLAND RB: Prevention of infection. *In:* Polk HC Jr (ed): Infection and the Surgical Patient. Edinburgh: Churchill Livingstone; 1982: 72–90.
4. CONDON RE: Intraluminal antibiotics. *In:* Polk HC Jr (ed): Infection and the Surgical Patient. Edinburgh: Churchill Livingstone; 1982: 62–71.
5. POLLOCK AV: Topical antibiotics. *In:* Polk HC Jr (ed): Infection and the Surgical Patient. Edinburgh: Churchill Livingstone; 1982: 91–100.
6. POLK HC Jr, LOPEZ-MAYOR JF: Postoperative wound infection: A prospective study of determinant factors and prevention. Surgery 1969;66:97.
7. BERNARD HR, COLE WR: The prophylaxis of surgical infection: The effect of prophylactic antimicrobial drugs on the incidence of infection following potentially contaminated operations. Surgery 1964;56:151.
8. NICHOLS RL, BROIDO P, CONDON RE et al: Effect of preoperative neomycin-erythromycin intestinal preparation on the incidence of infectious complications following colon surgery. Ann Surg 1973;178:453.
9. GORDON HE, GAYLOR DW, RICHMOND DM et al: Operations on the colon: The role of antibiotics in preoperative preparation. Calif Med 1965;103:243.
10. RUBBO SD, HUGHES ESR, BLAINEY B et al: Role of preoperative chemoprophylaxis in bowel surgery. Antimicrob Agents Chemother 1965;5:649.
11. EVERETT MT, BROGAN TD, NETTLETON J: The place of antibiotics in colonic surgery: A clinical study. Br J Surg 1969;56:679.
12. ROSENBERG IL, GRAHAM NG, De DOMBAL FT et al: Preparation of the intestine in patients undergoing major large-bowel surgery, mainly for neoplasms of the colon and rectum. Br J Surg 1971;58:266.

13. CLARKE JS, CONDON RE, BARTLETT JG et al: Preoperative oral antibiotics reduce septic complications of colon operations: Results of prospective, randomized, double-blind clinical study. Ann Surg 1977;186:251.

14. WASHINGTON JA II, DEARING WH, JUDD ES et al: Effect of preoperative antibiotic regimen on development of infection after intestinal surgery: Prospective, randomized, double-blind study. Ann Surg 1974;180, 567.

15. MATHESON DM, ARABI Y, BAXTER-SMITH D et al: Randomized multicentre trial of oral bowel preparation and antimicrobials for elective colorectal operations. Br J Surg 1978;65:597.

16. GOLDRING J, SCOTT A, McNAUGHT W et al: Prophylactic oral antimicrobial agents in elective colonic surgery. Lancet 1975;2:997.

17. PROUD G, CHAMBERLAIN J: Antimicrobial prophylaxis in elective colonic surgery. Lancet 1979;2:1017 (Letter).

18. HÖJER H, WETTERFORS J: Systemic prophylaxis with doxycycline in surgery of the colon and rectum. Ann Surg 1978;187:362.

19. BJERKESET T, DIGRANES A: Systemic prophylaxis with metronidazole (Flagyl) in elective surgery of the colon and rectum. Surgery 1980;87:560.

20. HUGHES ESR, HARDY KJ, CUTHBERTSON AM et al: Chemoprophylaxis in large bowel surgery. 1. Effect of intravenous administration of penicillin on incidence of postoperative infection. Med J Aust 1970;1:305.

21. BURTON RC, HUGHES ESR, CUTHBERTSON AM: Prophylactic use of gentamicin in colonic and rectal surgery. Med J Aust 1975;2:597.

22. KEIGHLEY MRB, CRAPP AR, BURDON DW et al: Prophylaxis against anaerobic sepsis in bowel surgery. Br J Surg 1976;63:538.

23. KJELLGREN K, SELLSTRÖM H: Effect of prophylactic systemic administration of cephalothin in colorectal surgery. Acta Chir Scand 1977;143:473.

24. FEATHERS RS, LEWIS AAM, SAGOR GR et al: Prophylactic systemic antibiotics in colorectal surgery. Lancet 1977;2:4.

25. BURDON JGW, MORRIS PJ, HUNT P et al: A trial of cephalothin sodium in colon surgery to prevent wound infection. Arch Surg 1977;112:1169.

26. GALLAND RB, SAUNDERS JH, MOSLEY JG et al: Prevention of wound infection in abdominal operations by peroperative antibiotics or povidone-iodine: A controlled trial. Lancet 1977;2:1043.

27. EYKYN SJ, JACKSON BT, LOCKHART-MUMMERY HE et al: Prophylactic peroperative intravenous metronidazole in elective colorectal surgery. Lancet 1979;2:761 (Letter).
28. CONDON RE, BARTLETT JG, NICHOLS RL et al: Preoperative prophylactic cephalothin fails to control septic complications of colorectal operations: Results of controlled clinical trial. Am J Surg 1979;137:68.
29. POLK HC Jr, TRACHTENBERG L, FINN MP: Antibiotic activity in surgical incisions: The basis for prophylaxis in selected operations. JAMA 1980;244:1353.
30. BAUM ML, ANISH DS, CHALMERS TC et al: A survey of clinical trials of antibiotic prophylaxis in colon surgery: Evidence against further use of no-treatment controls. N Engl J Med 1981;305:795.
31. PALMU A, RENKONEN O-V, AROMAA U: Ornidazole and anaerobic bacteria: In vitro sensitivity and effects on wound infections after appendectomy. J Infect Dis 1979;139:586.
32. ANDERSEN B, BENDTSEN A, HOLBRAAD L et al: Wound infections after appendicectomy. Acta Chir Scand 1972;138:531.
33. LEIGH DA, SIMMONS K, NORMAN E: Bacterial flora of the appendix fossa in appendicitis and postoperative wound infection. J Clin Pathol 1974;27:997.
34. RICKETT JWS, JACKSON BT: Topical ampicillin in the appendicectomy wound: Report of double-blind trial. Br Med J 1969;4:206.
35. GILMORE OJA, MARTIN TDM, FLETCHER BN: Prevention of wound infection after appendicectomy. Lancet 1973;1:220.
36. BATES L, DOWN RHL, HOUGHTON MCV et al: Topical ampicillin in the prevention of wound infection after appendicectomy. Br J Surg 1974;61:489.
37. WILLIS AT, FERGUSON IR, JONES PH et al: Metronidazole in prevention and treatment of bacteroides infection after appendicectomy. Br Med J 1976;1:318.
38. EVERSON NW, FOSSARD DP, NASH JR et al: Wound infection following appendicectomy: The effect of extraperitoneal wound drainage and systemic antibiotic prophylaxis. Br J Surg 1977;64:236.
39. FOSTER PD, O'TOOLE RD: Primary appendectomy: The effect of prophylactic cephaloridine on postoperative wound infection. JAMA 1978;239:1411.
40. GREENALL MJ, BAKRAN A, PICKFORD IR et al: A double-blind trial of a single intravenous dose of metronidazole as prophylaxis

against wound infection following appendicectomy. Br J Surg 1979;66:428.

41. DONOVAN IA, ELLIS D, GATEHOUSE D et al: One- dose antibiotic prophylaxis against wound infection after appendicectomy: A randomized trial of clindamycin, cefazolin sodium and a placebo. Br J Surg 1979;66:193.
42. GOTTRUP F: Prophylactic metronidazole in prevention of infection after appendicectomy: Report of a double-blind trial. Acta Chir Scand 1980;146:133.
43. BATES T, TOUQUET VLR, TUTTON MK et al: Prophylactic metronidazole in appendicectomy: A controlled trial. Br J Surg 1980;67:547.
44. FINE M, BUSUTTIL RW: Acute appendicitis: Efficacy of prophylactic preoperative antibiotics in the reduction of septic morbidity. Am J Surg 1978;135:210.
45. GRAY JDA, SHINER M: Influence of gastric pH on gastric and jejunal flora. Gut 1967;8:574.
46. DRASAR BS, SHINER M, McLEOD GM: Studies on the intestinal flora. I. The bacterial flora of the gastrointestinal tract in healthy and achlorhydric persons. Gastroenterology 1969;56:71.
47. GATEHOUSE D, DIMOCK F, BURDON DW et al: Prediction of wound sepsis following gastric operations. Br J Surg 1978; 65:551.
48. McKITTRICK LS, WHEELOCK FC Jr: The routine use of antibiotics in elective abdominal surgery. Surg Gynecol Obstet 1954; 99:376.
49. BARNES BA, BEHRINGER GE, WHEELOCK FC et al: Surgical sepsis: Report on subtotal gastrectomies. JAMA 1960;173:98.
50. SONNELAND J: Postoperative infection. II. Etiological factors. Pacif Med Surg 1966;74:165.
51. FELTIS JM Jr, HAMIT HF: Use of prophylactic antimicrobial drugs to prevent postoperative wound infections. Am J Surg 1967;114:867.
52. EVANS C, POLLOCK AV: The reduction of surgical wound infections by prophylactic parenteral cephaloridine: A controlled clinical trial. Br J Surg 1973;60:434.
53. GRIFFITHS DA, SHOREY BA, SIMPSON RA et al: Single-dose peroperative antibiotic prophylaxis in gastrointestinal surgery. Lancet 1976;2:325.
54. STONE HH, HOOPER CA, KOLB LD et al: Antibiotic prophylaxis in gastric, biliary and colonic surgery. Ann Surg 1976; 184:443.

55. LEWIS RT: Discriminate use of antibiotic prophylaxis in gastro-duodenal surgery. Am J Surg 1979;138:640.

56. PORIES WJ, VAN RIJ AM, BURLINGHAM BT et al: Prophylactic cefazolin in gastric bypass surgery. Surgery 1981;90:426.

57. STONE HH, HANEY BB, KOLB LD et al: Prophylactic and preventive antibiotic therapy: Timing, duration and economics. Ann Surg 1979;189:691.

58. ANDREWS E, HENRY LD: Bacteriology of normal and diseased gallbladders. Arch Intern Med 1935;133:1171.

59. EDLUND YA, MOLLSTEDT BO, OUCHTERLONY Ö: Bacteriological investigation of the biliary system and liver in biliary tract disease correlated to clinical data and microstructure of the gallbladder and liver. Acta Chir Scand 1958/1959; 116:461.

60. FLEMMA RJ, FLINT LM, OSTERHOUT S et al: Bacteriologic studies of biliary tract infection. Ann Surg 1967;166:563.

61. SCOTT AJ, KHAN GA: Origin of bacteria in bileduct bile. Lancet 1967;2:790.

62. CHETLIN SH, ELLIOTT DW: Biliary bacteremia. Arch Surg 1971;102:303.

63. ANDERSON RE, PRIESTLEY JT: Observations on the bacteriology of choledochal bile. Ann Surg 1951;133:486.

64. KEIGHLEY MRB, ALEXANDER-WILLIAMS J: Multivariate analysis of clinical and operative findings associated with biliary sepsis. Br J Surg 1976;63:528.

65. ELLIOTT DW: Biliary tract surgery. South Med J 1977;70, Suppl 1:31.

66. HALSALL AK, WELSH CL, CRAVEN JL et al: Prophylactic use of metronidazole in preventing wound sepsis after elective cholecystectomy. Br J Surg 1980;67:551.

67. STRACHAN CJL, BLACK J, POWIS SJA et al: Prophylactic use of cephazolin against wound sepsis after cholecystectomy. Br Med J 1977;1:1254.

68. BEVAN PG, WILLIAMS JD: Rifamide in acute cholecystitis and biliary surgery. Br Med J 1971;3:284.

69. KEIGHLEY MRB, DRYSDALE RB, QUORAISHI AH et al: Antibiotics in biliary disease: The relative importance of antibiotic concentrations in the bile and serum. Gut 1976;17:495.

70. KEIGHLEY MRB, BADDELEY RM, BURDON DW et al: A controlled trial of parenteral prophylactic gentamicin therapy in biliary surgery. Br J Surg 1975;62:275.

71. McLEISH AR, KEIGHLEY MRB, BISHOP HM et al: Selecting patients requiring antibiotics in biliary surgery by immediate gram stains of bile at operation. Surgery 1977;81:473.

72. ENGSTRÖM J, HELLSTRÖM K, HÖGMAN L et al: Microorganisms of the liver, biliary tract and duodenal aspirates in biliary diseases. Scand J Gastroenterol 1971;6:177.

73. CROTON RS, TREANOR J, GREEN HT et al: The evaluation of cefuroxime in the prevention of postoperative infection. Postgrad Med J 1981;57:363.

74. CUNHA BA, PYRTEK LJ, QUINTILIANI R: Prophylactic antibiotics in cholecystectomy. Lancet 1978;1:207 (Letter).

75. MATOLO NM, COHEN SE, WOLFMAN EF Jr: Effects of antibiotics on prevention of infection in contaminated abdominal operations. Am Surg 1976;42:123.

76. THADEPALLI H, GORBACH SL, BROIDO PW et al: Abdominal trauma, anaerobes, and antibiotics. Surg Gynecol Obstet 1973; 137:270.

77. BROCKENBROUGH EC, MOYLAN JA: Treatment of contaminated surgical wounds with a topical antibiotic: A double-blind study of 240 patients. Am Surg 1969;35:789.

78. FULLEN WD, HUNT J, ALTEMEIER WA: Prophylactic antibiotics in penetrating wounds of the abdomen. J Trauma 1972; 12:282.

79. CRENSHAW CA, GLANGES E, WEBBER CE et al: Cephalothin-tobramycin as a preventive antibiotic combination. Surg Gynecol Obstet 1978;147:713.

80. STONE HH, HESTER TR Jr: Incisional and peritoneal infection after emergency celiotomy. Am Surg 1973;177:669.

81. O'DONNELL VA, LOU MA, ALEXANDER JL et al: Role of antibiotics in penetrating abdominal trauma. Am Surg 1978;44:574.

82. O'DONNELL V, MANDAL AK, LOU MA et al: Evaluation of carbenicillin and a comparison of clindamycin and gentamicin combined therapy in penetrating abdominal trauma. Surg Gynecol Obstet 1978;147:525.

83. POLK HC Jr, FINN MF: Chemoprophylaxis and immunoprophylaxis in surgical wound infection. In: Simmons RL, Howard RJ (eds): Surgical Infectious Disease. New York: Appleton-Century-Crofts, 1982.

84. ALTEMEIER WA: Cited in Discussion. In: Washington JA II, Dearing WH, Judd ES et al.[14]

Chapter 3

THORACIC SURGERY

In a multicenter study on the effectiveness of ultraviolet light in the operating room, the rate of wound infection reported after 388 clean thoracotomies was 5.7%.[1] In a review of 857 clean thoracotomies performed at one hospital during a 28-month period, Nelson and Nelson[2] reported only 5 wound infections (0.6%). They suggested that the extraordinarily low infection rate may have been due in part to the use of antibiotic prophylaxis in almost all (97%) of the patients.

The effectiveness of antibiotic prophylaxis in thoracic surgery was given further support in an uncontrolled study reported by Bryant et al.[3] In a retrospective analysis for the year 1972, they reported an incidence of 18.4% for wound infection and empyema associated with "inadequate or irregular administration of prophylactic antibiotics." In 1973, after instituting a "standard regimen" of preoperative and postoperative administration of cephalothin and cephalexin for 3 days and wound irrigation with cephalothin and kanamycin, the "infectious complication" rate was decreased to 4.8%.

Five well-designed controlled trials[4-8] of antibiotic prophylaxis in thoracic surgery were subsequently reported. In three of these reports, the investigators[4,7,8] concluded that antibiotic prophylaxis was of value; in two reports, the investigators[5,6] concluded that it was not.

In a prospective double-blind study by Kvale et al.,[4] 77 patients who had elective pulmonary resections were given either placebo or cefazolin preoperatively and every 6 hours after surgery or until oral medication could be tolerated. Cephalexin was given for 5 days postoperatively. Primary bronchogenic carcinoma was the most common diagnosis for which surgery was performed (42 of 77 patients). Major infections were defined as pneumonia, wound or chest-wall abscess, empyema, purulent bronchitis, bacteremia, and infection of the urinary tract. Wound cellulitis without purulent discharge and mucocutaneous infections were defined as minor (Table 3–1). The overall infection rate in the antibiotic group was 19% and

Table 3–1. Antibiotic Prophylaxis in Pulmonary Resection

Infection	Antibiotic Group (N = 43)		Placebo Group (N = 34)		p Value
Major infections					
Pneumonia	1	(2.3%)	9	(26%)	= 0.004
Purulent bronchitis	1	(2.3%)	0		NS
Empyema and wound abscess	0		5	(15%)	= 0.028
Total major infections	3	(7%)	14*	(41%)	= 0.0006
Minor infections	5†	(12%)	3	(9%)	NS
Total of all infections	8	(19%)	17	(50%)	= 0.005

* 11 patients with 14 infections.
† 4 patients with 5 infections.
N, number of patients; NS, not significant.
Modified from data of Kvale et al.,[4] with permission.

Table 3–2. Infection Rate According to the Extent of Pulmonary Resection

Type of Surgery (No. of Patients)	Major Infections No. (%)	Minor Infections No. (%)	Total No. of Infections No. (%)
Pneumonectomy (11)	3 (27)	1 (9)	4 (36)
Lobectomy (37)	7 (19)	6 (16)	13 (35)
Wedge resection lung plus pleural biopsy; bullectomy (29)	7 (24)	1 (3)	8 (28)
p values	NS	NS	NS

NS, not significant.
From Kvale et al.,[4] with permission.

was 50% in the placebo group. The minor infection rates, 12% and 9% in the antibiotic and placebo groups, respectively, were not significantly different. Thus, reduction in major infection was the principal effect observed in the antibiotic group.

Further analysis of the data[4] showed that the reduction in major infection attributable to prophylaxis was due to a marked decrease in the incidence of pneumonia (from 26% to 2.3%) and empyema and wound abscess (from 15% to 0). In this trial, the extent of pulmonary resection had no effect on the incidence of infection (Table 3–2). One patient in the placebo group died 6 weeks after surgery, apparently of a pulmonary embolus. There were no other deaths in either group.

Truesdale et al.[5] conducted a similar double-blind prospective study of 57 patients undergoing noncardiac thoracic surgical procedures. Cefazolin was administered preoperatively and cephalothin postoperatively for 48 hours. Infection was not clearly defined. Lobectomy and pneumonectomy were defined as major procedures; wedge resection and exploratory thoracotomy without resection were defined as minor procedures.

There was no significant difference in the overall infection rate between the placebo group (17.2%) and the prophylaxis group (17.8%) (Table 3–3). When the patients were grouped according to the extent of surgery, there were still no significant differences. Analysis of other indices of infection, such as the white blood cell count, fever, and duration of hospital stay, revealed no significant difference between the placebo and prophylaxis groups. Moreover, complications of prophylaxis occurred in 5 of 29 (17.2%) and 18 of 28 (64.4%) patients in the placebo and prophylaxis groups, respectively ($p < 0.001$) (Table 3–4). Five deaths associated with infection

Table 3–3. Postoperative Rates of Infection

Category	No.	%
All study patients		
Placebo	5/29	17.2
Cefazolin/cephalothin	5/28	17.8
Major procedures		
Placebo	5/20	25.0
Cefazolin/cephalothin	4/23	17.4
Minor procedures		
Placebo	0/9	0
Cefazolin/cephalothin	1/5	20.0

From Truesdale et al.,[5] with permission.

Table 3–4. Undesirable Effects Induced by Administration of Cefazolin/Cephalothin Prophylaxis

Undesirable Effect	Cefazolin/Cephalothin		Placebo		Statistical Significance
	No.	%	No.	%	
Hypersensitivity reactions	1/28	3.6	1/29	3.4	NS
Drug fever	7/28	25.0	2/29	6.8	$0.025 < p < 0.05$
Phlebitis	10/27	37.0	2/28	7.1	$p < 0.005$
Elevated BUN level	4/25	16.0	0/23	0	$0.01 < p < 0.025$
Abnormal liver-function study values	2/17	11.7	2/27	7	NS

NS, not significant.
From Truesdale et al.,[5] with permission.

occurred in the study; 2 of the patients had received the cephalo-sporin prophylaxis and 3 had received placebo.

Thus, Truesdale et al.[5] were unable to show any benefit of prophylaxis; in fact, they reported an increase in cephalosporin-related side effects in the prophylaxis group. There were important differences between their study and the study of Kvale et al.[4]: (1) Kvale et al. noted a 50% incidence of infection in their placebo group, as compared with 17.2% in the study of Truesdale et al.[5]; (2) infection rates were the same regardless of the extent of surgery in the report by Kvale et al., whereas almost all the infections reported by Truesdale et al. occurred in patients undergoing major surgery.

Cameron et al.[6] conducted a larger but similar investigation. The trial was randomized and prospective, but not double-blind. Patients in the prophylaxis group were given cephalothin before, during, and after surgery for a total of four doses. The control group was given no antibiotic. The study included 171 patients, 83 in the control group and 88 in the prophylaxis group. Criteria for infection were not clearly stated. In 136 of 177 patients, pulmonary resection was performed for malignant disease.

"Septic complications" occurred in 23 of 83 patients in the control group and in 16 of 88 patients in the prophylaxis group.[6] These differences were not significant ($p > 0.1$). In addition, there were no significant differences when septic complications were analyzed separately, for example, pneumonia, empyema, wound infection, or bronchopleural fistula, or when the groups were compared for duration of postoperative stay or fever. Two patients in the study died, both in the prophylaxis group. The authors reported that "there were no recognized complications or allergic reactions secondary to cephalothin administration." However, the method used to detect adverse reactions was not described. An increase in gram-negative infection was noted in those patients receiving cephalosporin prophylaxis.

Thus, the negative observations of Cameron et al.[6] appear to confirm those of Truesdale et al.[5] and to contradict those of Kvale et al.[4]

A larger double-blind study[7] (211 patients) appeared to reach a middle ground in assessing the value of antibiotic prophylaxis in noncardiac thoracic surgery. In this trial, 118 patients received cephalothin immediately preoperatively and at 4 hours postoperatively; 91 patients received placebo. Infection criteria were carefully defined. Lobectomy was the most common operation performed; gastric (hiatus hernia) surgery and esophageal surgery were the next most common.

Postoperative wound infection was significantly reduced in the prophylaxis group, but not pulmonary infection or empyema (Table 3–5). Two deaths occurred in the prophylaxis group (1.7%) and 4 in the placebo group (4.3%). This difference was not significant.

No direct toxic effects of cephalothin prophylaxis were described, although it is not clear whether they were systematically sought. Ilves et al.[7] observed that the short-term prophylaxis used in their study did not contribute to bacterial resistance, since 15 of the 17 pulmonary infections in the antibiotic group were due to cephalothin-sensitive organisms.

Unlike Kvale et al.[4] these investigators did not show that deep infection, such as pneumonia and empyema, was prevented by prophylaxis. On the other hand, and contrary to the observations of Truesdale et al.[5] and Cameron et al.,[6] the incidence of wound infection was reduced in the prophylaxis group. Ilves et al.[7] concluded their report by recommending the use of antibiotic prophylaxis in most thoracotomies, which they regarded as "clean-contaminated" rather than "clean" surgery.

In a recent controlled trial,[8] short-term high-dose penicillin prophylaxis was compared with placebo. The rate of wound infection, postoperative antibiotic use, and postoperative hospital stay were reduced in the penicillin group. Prophylaxis had no effect on the incidence of lower respiratory infection or empyema. The authors observed an increase in respiratory tract colonization and postoperative infections with Enterobacteriaceae and *Pseudomonas aeruginosa* in the penicillin group.

In a retrospective analysis of the treatment of spontaneous pneumothorax with tube thoracostomy or pleural abrasion (or both), Neugebauer et al.[9] concluded that the duration of hospitalization was longer in the prophylaxis group and that the incidence of "complications" and drug reactions was higher as well. Criteria for

Table 3–5. Prophylaxis of Incisional Infection

	Total Cases	Wound Infections		Pulmonary Infections	Empyema
		Deep	Superficial		
Cephalothin	118	1 (0.8%)	6 (5.1%)	17 (14.4%)	5 (4.2%)
Placebo	93	5 (5.4%)	17 (18.3%)	25 (26.9%)	6 (6.5%)

From Ilves et al.,[7] with permission.

Table 3-6. Clinical Characteristics of Patients Sustaining Thoracic Trauma

	Type of Injury	Hemothorax	Pneumothorax	Chest Tube Drainage (ml)	Chest Tube Duration (days)	Drug Treatment (days)	Follow-Up (%)
Clindamycin group N = 38	14 GSW 24 SW	25	31	646	5.0	4.7	87
Placebo group N = 37	10 GSW 27 SW	29	31	565	5.2	5.1	87

GSW, gunshot wound; SW, stab wound.
Modified from Grover et al.,[10] with permission.

infection, detailed microbiologic information, and the types and duration of antibiotics used for prophylaxis were omitted from their report. Methodologic and other flaws impair analysis of this report and render it nonevaluable.

On the basis of experience and investigation of antibiotic prophylaxis in abdominal and orthopedic trauma, one might expect that prophylaxis would be useful in managing patients with penetrating chest trauma. In a prospective double-blind study of 75 patients with gunshot wounds or stab wounds of the chest, Grover et al.[10] showed this to be the case (Table 3–6). Thirty-eight patients received clindamycin phosphate intravenously every 6 hours until 1 day after removal of the chest tube, or for 5 days, whichever was the shorter period. Thirty-seven patients received placebo. Roentgenographically documented pneumonia was more common in the placebo group (13/37) than in the antibiotic group (4/38). This difference was statistically significant ($p < 0.03$). The incidences of empyema, elevated white blood cell counts, fever, and wound infection, and the incidence of positive pleural cultures were all less in the prophylaxis group than in the placebo group. However, because of the small number of patients in each group, the differences did not achieve statistical significance. The authors terminated the study prematurely because of increasing reports of clindamycin-associated colitis in the literature, although none of the patients in their trial experienced this adverse effect. Various gram-positive and gram-negative organisms were isolated from wound and sputum cultures. Because precise definitions of infection were not included in the methods, it is unclear which of the organisms were infective and which were normal or transient flora.

MICROBIOLOGIC CONSIDERATIONS

In three[4,6,8] of the five trials described,[4-8] the authors presented detailed information on the organisms causing infection and their antibiotic sensitivities. Table 3–7 shows that in the series reported by Kvale et al.,[4] many different gram-positive and gram-negative organisms caused postoperative infection in the placebo and prophylaxis groups. Thus, a clear-cut effect of cephalosporin administration on the microbiology of infection was not demonstrated. No anaerobes were reported as having been isolated from this group of infected patients.

Table 3–7. Infections Listed by Diagnosis, Severity, and Bacteriologic Findings

Patient	Type of Infection	Severity	Organisms Recovered
		Antibiotic Group	
1	Bacteremia	Major	*Herellea* sp.
2	Pneumonia	Major	*Streptococcus pneumoniae*
3	Purulent bronchitis	Major	*Haemophilus influenzae*
4	Cellulitis	Minor	——
5	Herpes labialis and	Minor	——
	Inguinal cutaneous candidiasis	Minor	*Candida*
6	Cellulitis	Minor	——
7	Cellulitis	Minor	——
		Placebo Group	
1	Pneumonia and	Major	*H. influenzae*
	Empyema	Major	*Staphylococcus aureus*
2	Wound abscess	Major	α-Hemolytic *Streptococcus* and *Staphylococcus epidermidis*
3	Pneumonia	Major	——
4	(a) Pneumonia	Major	*H. influenzae*
	(b) Wound abscess	Major	*S. aureus*
5	Empyema	Major	*S. aureus*
6	Pneumonia	Major	*S. pneumoniae* *S. aureus* *H. influenzae*
7	Pneumonia	Major	*Pseudomonas aeruginosa*
8	(a) Pneumonia and	Major	*S. aureus*
	(b) Empyema	Major	*S. aureus*
9	Pneumonia	Major	——
10	Pneumonia	Major	*Proteus mirabilis* *S. pneumoniae*
11	Pneumonia	Major	*S. pneumoniae* and *S. aureus*
12	Cellulitis	Minor	——
13	Cellulitis	Minor	——
14	Cellulitis	Minor	——

From Kvale et al.,[4] with permission.

In contrast, Cameron et al.[6] concluded that three doses of perioperative cephalothin shifted the cause of postoperative infection from gram-positive (largely sensitive) organisms to gram-negative organisms, half of which were resistant to cephalothin

(Table 3–8). It is important to note that in this series of patients, topical intraoperative irrigation with neomycin and polymyxin was used in addition to the systemic cephalothin prophylaxis (or placebo). Since these additional antibiotics were used in all patients, their effect on the incidence or bacteriology of postoperative infection is unknown. Similarly, Frimodt-Møller et al.[8] observed that perioperative penicillin (5,000,000 units for 6 doses) resulted in an increased rate of respiratory colonization with resistant gram-negative rods.

PRACTICAL RECOMMENDATIONS

Double-blind prospective trials have provided conflicting data in elective noncardiac thoracic surgery, and therefore firm recommendations cannot be made. One can find support in the literature for

Table 3–8. Organisms Identified in Postoperative Infections in Thoracic Surgery Patients Receiving Cephalothin

Organisms	Control, No.		Antibiotic, No.	
Gram-positive				
Staphylococcus aureus	12		3	
α-*Streptococcus*	3		4	
Pneumococcus	2		1	
Clostridium	1		——	
Staphylococcus epidermidis	1		——	
Streptococcus group D	1		1	
Total	20		9	
Gram-negative				
Klebsiella	——		6	
Proteus	1		6	
Escherichia coli	1		4	
Enterobacteriaceae	2		4	
Pseudomonas	1		4	
Bacteroides fragilis	——		1	
Neisseria	1		——	
Haemophilus influenzae	2		——	
Haemophilus parainfluenzae	3		1	
Total	11		26	
Sensitivities	S	R	S	R
	20	6	16	18

S, sensitive; R, resistant.
From Cameron et al.,[6] with permission.

either using or not using antibiotic prophylaxis. If it is used, short-term cefazolin prophylaxis (3 doses given perioperatively) is recommended to lessen toxicity, cost, and the effect on the patient's normal flora.

Single-dose preoperative prophylaxis with newer long half-life cephalosporins may be feasible, but requires confirmation by controlled trials. Data are inadequate to support a recommendation for prophylaxis in the management of spontaneous pneumothorax; we therefore advise against using antibiotics in this situation unless signs or symptoms of infection are present. Antibiotics are indicated in the management of patients with penetrating chest trauma; this use should be categorized as therapeutic rather than prophylactic.

REFERENCES

1. NATIONAL ACADEMY OF SCIENCES–NATIONAL RESEARCH COUNCIL: Postoperative wound infection. Report of Ad Hoc Committee of Committee on Trauma. Ann Surg 1964; 160:332.

2. NELSON JC, NELSON RM: The incidence of hospital wound infection in thoracotomies. J Thorac Cardiovasc Surg 1967; 54:586.

3. BRYANT LR, DILLON ML, MOBIN-UDDIN K: Prophylactic antibiotics in noncardiac thoracic operations. Ann Thorac Surg 1975;19:670.

4. KVALE PA, RANGA V, KOPACZ M et al: Pulmonary resection. South Med J 1977;70, Suppl 1:64.

5. TRUESDALE R, D'ALESSANDRI R, MANUEL V et al: Antimicrobial vs placebo prophylaxis in noncardiac thoracic surgery. JAMA 1979;241:1254.

6. CAMERON JL, IMBEMBO A, KIEFFER RF et al: Prospective clinical trial of antibiotics for pulmonary resections. Surg Gynecol Obstet 1981;152:156.

7. ILVES R, COOPER JD, TODD TRJ et al: Prospective, randomized, double-blind study using prophylactic cephalothin for major, elective, general thoracic operations. J Thorac Cardiovasc Surg 1981;81:813.

8. FRIMODT-MØLLER N, OSTRI P, PEDERSON IK et al: Antibiotic prophylaxis in pulmonary surgery. Ann Surg 1982;195:444.

9. NEUGEBAUER MK, FOSBURG RG, TRUMMER MJ: Routine antibiotic therapy following pleural space intubation. J Thorac Cardiovasc Surg 1971;61:882.

10. GROVER FL, RICHARDSON JD, FEWEL JG et al: Prophylactic antibiotics in the treatment of penetrating chest wounds: A prospective double-blind study. J Thorac Cardiovasc Surg 1977;74:528.

Chapter 4

CARDIAC SURGERY

CLINICAL STUDIES

Historically, cardiac surgery can be viewed as similar to other surgical specialties with respect to evaluation of antibiotic prophylaxis. Closed cardiac surgery, without cardiopulmonary bypass, is intrinsically a low-risk, clean operation,[1] and one would today anticipate little protection by systemic antibiotics.

The era of "open-heart" surgery and the pump-oxygenator brought with it high postoperative infection rates and some mortality associated with infection. In a retrospective analysis of 222 patients who underwent surgery between 1957 and 1960, Kittle and Reed[2] reported postoperative infection rates of 3.5% and 22% in "closed" and "open-heart" surgical cases, respectively. Almost half of the infections in the open-heart group were bacteremias. Coagulase-negative and coagulase-positive staphylococci were the preponderant organisms. Infection rates in the group receiving prophylaxis (various combinations of penicillin, streptomycin, chloramphenicol, tetracycline, and erythromycin) and the group receiving no prophylaxis were not significantly different (Table 4–1). Thus, the authors concluded that prophylactic antibiotics were of no value in this group of patients. Although this study is important from a historical standpoint, it must be noted that it was uncontrolled, no standard antibiotic regimen was used, and antibiotics were given postoperatively.

Lord et al.[3] reported their own experience and data summarized from questionnaires addressed to 12 surgical teams performing "open-heart" procedures: a 2.2% incidence (7 infections in 315 patients) of endocarditis in patients receiving preoperative prophylaxis and an 0.5% incidence (11 infections in 2,170 patients) of endocarditis in patients not receiving postoperative prophylaxis. Thus, these authors concluded that preoperative antibiotic prophylaxis might actually favor the development of postoperative endocarditis.

Table 4-1. Early Studies of Antibiotic Prophylaxis in Cardiac Surgery

Procedure	Total No. of Patients	No Prophylactic Antibiotics Given			Prophylactic Antibiotics		
		No. of Patients	No Infection	Infection	No. of Patients	No Infection	Infection
Repair of coarctation of aorta	18	11	11	0	7	7	0
Transsection of ductus arteriosus	41	21	21	0	20	20	0
Mitral valvotomy	55	25	21	4	30	30	0
Extracorporeal circulation	108	62	48	14*	46	36	10†
Total	222						

* Two deaths.
† Five deaths.

From Kittle and Reed,[2] with permission.

Table 4-2. Infections Related to Prophylactic Antibiotic Regimens

Therapeutic Group	Number of Patients	Total No. of Infected Patients	Classification of Infections			
			Major	Wound	Urinary Tract	Pulmonary
Placebo	15	5	2	3	2	1
Penicillin + streptomycin	30	8	2	2	4	2
Oxacillin	27	7	3	1	4	1
Total	72	20	7	6	10	4

From Goodman et al,[14] with permission.

Investigators[4] studying 93 consecutive patients (94 procedures) undergoing open-heart surgery in the early 1960s came to the opposite conclusion. In 16 patients who received no prophylaxis there were 7 infections (5 bacteremias); in 35 patients who received postoperative prophylaxis there were 7 infections (7 bacteremias); in 43 patients who received preoperative prophylaxis there were 2 infections (2 bacteremias).

Of 14 infections for which a causative agent was identified, 11 (79%) were due to *Staphylococcus aureus* or "*Staphylococcus albus.*" Three of the 14 (21%) infections were due to "Pseudomonas" (1 in the "no antibiotic" group and 2 in the "preoperative antibiotic" group). The authors[4] concluded that preoperative prophylaxis was useful in patients undergoing open-heart surgery.

This report too is of historical importance, because it again documented the high infection rates associated with open-heart surgery and raised the possibility that preoperative administration of antibiotics may be necessary to achieve a favorable effect. However, controls were not concurrent or randomized, and multiple antibiotic regimens (penicillin, streptomycin, chloramphenicol, erythromycin, vancomycin, ristocetin, kanamycin, tetracycline) were used.

After these early reports, a number of retrospective reviews were published, all of which emphasized the importance of prophylactic antibiotics to prevent infectious endocarditis associated with cardiac surgery.[5-11] Despite these studies, the emergence of resistant organisms[12] and fungi[13] in patients receiving prophylaxis, and the lack of convincing controlled data confirming efficacy, encouraged controversy about the role of antibiotic prophylaxis in cardiac surgery. The first randomized placebo-controlled prospective trial of antibiotic prophylaxis for cardiac surgery was reported in 1968 by Goodman et al.[14] The study comprised 72 patients, 41 with and 31 without cardiopulmonary bypass. Patients were placed on one of three regimens: placebo; or 1.5 million units of penicillin and 250 mg of streptomycin every 6 hours; or oxacillin, 1 g, every 6 hours. Each regimen was begun on the morning of surgery and continued for 3 days (Table 4–2).

The placebo group was terminated when 2 patients suffered pneumococcal endocarditis. Two major infections (one coagulase-positive and penicillin-resistant and the other coagulase-negative and penicillin-resistant) occurred in the penicillin-streptomycin group. Three major infections (one oxacillin-sensitive, one oxacillin-resistant, and one unknown) occurred in the oxacillin group.

Goodman et al. concluded that none of the three regimens appeared superior with regard to major or minor infection, that prophylaxis may have selected for antibiotic-resistant strains, and that the onset of major infections may have been delayed by prophylactic antibiotic administration. Again, in this study, the high rate of infection (41%) was noted in patients undergoing cardiopulmonary bypass.

Fekety et al.[15] studied 213 patients undergoing cardiac surgery in 1963 and 1964. Although the study was prospective, it was not randomized or double-blind. Their "no prophylaxis" group included only patients having surgery without cardiopulmonary bypass. In this series, methicillin was not shown to be superior to penicillin prophylaxis. The authors noted that while staphylococcal infections were less frequent in the methicillin group, gram-negative organisms (*Klebsiella* sp. and unspecified others) were responsible for 6 of 7 infections in these patients. All 14 bacterial species isolated in this series were sensitive to cephalothin. Ten of the 213 patients (4.7%) experienced urticarial or maculopapular skin eruptions. The incidence of these reactions was not significantly different among the three groups. These authors concluded their study by expressing doubt about the efficacy of prophylaxis for cardiac surgery; they suggested that other antibiotics, particularly cephalothin, be evaluated.

In 1972, Conte et al.[16] published the results of a prospective randomized double-blind study comparing single-dose with multiple-dose cephalothin prophylaxis in patients undergoing cardiopulmonary bypass. The multiple-dose group received cephalothin, 1 g, intravenously every 6 hours, beginning the evening before surgery and continuing for a total of 20 doses. The single-dose group received 20 doses of placebo on the same schedule. All patients received 1 g of cephalothin intraoperatively during cardiopulmonary bypass.

There were no significant differences between the multiple-dose group and the single-dose group when compared for rates of major and minor infection, mortality, and floral changes (Table 4–3). Although the authors[16] suggested that a shift to resistant gram-negative major infection occurred in the multiple-dose group, this observation was not confirmed in a subsequent study[17] in which the authors concluded that single-dose intraoperative prophylaxis was as effective as a multiple-dose prophylactic regimen.

A larger study comparing 6-day and 2-day regimens of cephalothin prophylaxis was reported by Goldmann et al.[17] This trial was also prospective, randomized, and double-blind. Patients in the 2-day group were given 1 g of cephalothin intravenously on call to the

Table 4–3. Summary of Infections, Deaths (with or without Infection), and Floral Changes

Criterion	No. in Multiple-Dose Group	No. in Single-Dose Group	Total	Percent
Satisfy conditions of protocol	34	30	64	100
Patients with major infection(s)*	5	6	11	17
Patients with minor infection(s)*	8	9	17	27
Deaths in hospital with infection*	0	1	1	1.5
Deaths in hospital without infection*	1	1	2	3.1
Floral changes*†	21	13	34	53
Floral changes of consequence*	3	5	8	12

* No significant differences between multiple-dose and single-dose groups (p > 0.20).

† No significant differences among groups when floral changes were subcategorized into respiratory or stool changes or both.

From Conte JE Jr et al.,[16] with permission.

Table 4-4. Infection Rates in Patients Receiving Protocol Antibiotic for More Than 2 Days

Site	6-Day Group		2-Day Group		Total	
	No.	%	No.	%	No.	%
Pneumonia	9	8.5	5	5.3	14	7.0
Bronchitis	0	0	2	2.1	2	1.0
Urinary tract infection	9	8.5	16	17.0	25	12.5
Sternal wound	3	2.8	2	2.1	5	2.5
Other wound	2	1.9	1	1.1	3	1.5
Bacteremia associated with infection at another site	4	3.8	4	4.3	8	4.0
Bacteremia not associated with infection at another site	0	0	0	0	0	0
Total number of infections	27	25.5	30	31.9	57	28.5
Total number of infected patients	16	15.1	23	24.5	39	19.5

From Goldmann et al.,[17] with permission.

operating room, 2 g intravenously during bypass, and then 2 g intravenously every 6 hours for 7 more doses. Patients in the 6-day group were placed on the same schedule except that the cephalothin every 6 hours was continued for 23 doses (6 days). Rates of major and minor infection were not significantly different in the 2-day and 6-day groups (Table 4–4). Cephalothin appeared to prevent catheter-associated urinary tract infections during antibiotic administration. However, fungal and antibiotic-resistant urinary tract infections were more common in the 6-day than in the 2-day group. The reverse was true for pneumonia, but the difference was not statistically significant. Wound infections and 2 bacteremias were equally distributed between the two study groups. There were no cases of endocarditis. The authors concluded that cephalothin prophylaxis was of value in prosthetic valve surgery and that a 6-day period of administration was not superior to a 2-day period.

Kini et al.[18] compared cefazolin and cephalothin prophylaxis for patients undergoing cardiopulmonary bypass. The study was prospective, double-blind, and randomized; antibiotics were administered before, during, and after operation for 5 days. Three of 92 evaluable patients (3.3%) had postoperative infections, 1 in the cefazolin group and 2 in the cephalothin group. These differences were not significant. There were no cases of endocarditis. Three of the original 99 patients (3%) were dropped from the analysis because a rash precluded continuation of the protocol drug (cephalothin group). No anaphylactic reactions occurred. Because infection rates in this report were low, the authors were cautious in interpreting their data. They concluded that cefazolin appeared to be as effective and safe as cephalothin for prophylaxis during cardiac surgery.

Muers et al.[19] conducted a prospective but not blind trial of benzylpenicillin and flucloxacillin prophylaxis versus no treatment for 431 patients undergoing cardiac pacemaker implantation. They reported that antibiotic prophylaxis reduced their postoperative "generator pocket" infection rate from 3.6% to 0.9%.

MICROBIOLOGIC CONSIDERATIONS

Gram-negative rods are the preponderant pathogens associated with pneumonia and urinary tract infection in patients receiving cephalothin prophylaxis (Table 4–5).

The source of antibiotic-resistant *Staphylococcus epidermidis* in patients undergoing cardiac surgery has been investigated by

Table 4–5. Causes of Postoperative Infections in Patients Receiving
Cephalothin Prophylaxis for Cardiac Surgery

Cause of Infection	No. of Isolates	Day of Onset	Cephalothin Resistance
Pneumonia			
6-day group			
E. coli	3	2-3	1 resistant
K. pneumoniae	3	2-4	All sensitive
H. influenzae	2	2	Not tested
Other	2	3-4	All resistant
2-day group			
A. calcoaceticus	3	3-6	All resistant
H. influenzae	2	2-6	Not tested
Other	2	3-30	All resistant
In study less than 2 days			
Multiple coliforms	4	5-6	1/4 sensitive
Urinary tract infection			
6-day group			
Enterococcus	3	12-16	Multiple resistance
Candida sp.	2	9-29	Not tested
Other	4	8-11	Multiple resistance
2-day group			
E. coli	12	4-18	1 resistant
Other	6	4-16	3/3 tested were resistant

From data of Goldmann et al.,[17] with permission.

Table 4–6. Methicillin Susceptibility of *Staphylococcus
epidermidis* Isolates Recovered from Chests of
Cardiac Surgery Patients

Source of Isolate	Subpopulations Resistant to Methicillin concentration of*	
	12.5 μg/ml	100 μg/ml
Preoperative chest	13/55 (24)	3/55 (5.5)
Postoperative wound	33/55 (64)	29/55 (53)

*Number of patients with resistant isolates/number of patients sampled. Numbers
in parentheses are percentages.
From Archer and Tenenbaum,[20] with permission.

Archer and Tenenbaum.[20] The authors cultured specimens from the
chests of 80 patients before and after surgery. Prophylactic antibiotic
regimens consisted of various combinations of nafcillin, penicillin,
streptomycin, cephalothin, and cefamandole. The recovery of
methicillin-resistant *S. epidermidis* was markedly increased in postoperative chest cultures (Table 4–6). In addition, these organisms

Table 4–7. Antimicrobial Resistance to Selected Antibiotics of
Staphylococcus epidermidis Isolates from Cardiac Surgery
Patients

Concentration (μg/ml)	Source of Isolates*	
of Antibiotic in Agar	Preoperative	Postoperative
Methicillin (100)	0/30 (0)†	30/30 (100)
Nafcillin (100)	0/30 (0)	30/30 (100)
Cephalothin (25)	0/30 (0)	28/30 (93)
Cefamandole (25)	1/30 (3)	24/30 (80)
Penicillin (1.6)	4/30 (13)	30/30 (100)
Streptomycin (100)	3/30 (10)	20/30 (67)
Gentamicin (5)	0/30 (0)	6/30 (20)

*Isolates are preoperative (methicillin-susceptible) and 5 days postoperative (methicillin-
resistant) pairs from the chests of 30 patients.
† Number of isolates resistant/number of isolates tested. Numbers in parentheses are
percentages.
From Archer and Tenenbaum,[20] with permission.

were resistant to many commonly used antibiotics (Table 4–7). This finding suggests that antibiotic-resistant *S. epidermidis,* organisms that cause prosthetic valve endocarditis, may be hospital-acquired and, further, that these organisms are acquired perioperatively. The implications of these observations with regard to the selection of antibiotic prophylaxis and the prevention of endocarditis are uncertain and require further investigation.

PHARMACOLOGIC CONSIDERATIONS

It is important to have an antibiotic concentration at the site of potential bacterial contamination sufficient to prevent bacterial implantation and infection, either on the valve or in the valve-suture line.

Archer et al.[21] investigated aspects of antibiotic prophylaxis that might prevent prosthetic valve infection. Comparing cephalothin with cefamandole in a randomized prospective study, they concluded that both agents have similar activity against staphylococci. They also studied antibiotic concentrations in plasma before and during cardiopulmonary bypass, antibiotic concentrations in cardiac tissue, and the effect of prophylaxis on the incidence of postoperative infections. When administered in the operating room during induction of anesthesia, both agents achieved plasma antibiotic concentrations in excess (> 20 ug/ml) of the minimal inhibitory concentration of most staphylococci and diphtheroids.[21] Cefamandole and cephalothin levels fell less than 25% during a mean of 2 hours on cardiopulmonary bypass.

Williams and Steele[22] had previously demonstrated that the elimination of cephalothin was markedly slowed after cardiopulmonary bypass was begun. Valve and atrial appendage concentrations of cefamandole were three to five times higher than those of cephalothin. They suggested that this difference was related to physicochemical characteristics of the cefamandole molecule, such as pKa and lipophilia. From these data they concluded that cefamandole may be a better antibiotic for prophylaxis during cardiac surgery. However, this has not been confirmed by a controlled clinical trial.

Pien et al.[23] compared the effectiveness of clindamycin and cephalothin in patients undergoing cardiac surgery. There were no significant differences in the overall frequency of postoperative infections in these two antibiotic groups. Wound infection developed more frequently in the cephalothin group, whereas urinary tract infection was more common in the clindamycin group. Although clindamycin is inhibitory for both *S. aureus* and *S. epidermidis,* it is not bactericidal for these organisms.

In their review of patients undergoing cardiac surgery, Hirschmann and Inui[24] concluded that antibiotic prophylaxis should not exceed 48 hours. Further, they postulated that adequate serum antibiotic concentrations need to be maintained only for the duration of the operation.

In one controlled study, single-dose intraoperative prophylaxis was as effective as a multiple-dose regimen.[16] On this basis, short-term perioperative prophylaxis is recommended for cardiac surgery. Single-dose preoperative administration of drugs with a long half-life such as cefazolin, ceforanide, cefonicid, or ceftriaxone may be effective, but this method requires further careful investigation before it can be routinely recommended.

SURGICAL CONSIDERATIONS

The factors that predispose to prosthetic valve endocarditis are intraoperative bacteremia, often secondary to contamination of the coronary bypass equipment; postoperative bacteremias associated with intravenous catheters; infection of the operative wound or urinary or respiratory tract; and a foreign body in the heart.

Two basic types of valve prosthesis are commonly used: the totally artificial plastic and metal (mechanical) valve and the bioprosthetic valve that combine autologous, homologous, or heterologous tissue with a cloth-covered supporting strut. Oyer et al.[25] documented the superiority of glutaraldehyde-preserved porcine heterograft valves over Starr-Edwards valves with respect to thromboembolic phenomenon, hemorrhagic complications, and long-term survival. In addition, it has been suggested that patients with tissue valves are less likely to have prosthetic valve endocarditis, perivalvular abscesses, and periprosthetic leaks after the onset of infection.[26–28] Oyer et al.[25] postulated that tissue valves have an advantage over mechanical valves because they can be more easily sterilized with antimicrobial therapy after the onset of infection.

Rossiter et al.,[29] in a study of 2,184 patients who underwent either isolated aortic valve replacement or mitral valve replacement (1,347 Starr-Edwards valves and 837 glutaraldehyde-preserved porcine bioprosthetic heterografts), reported that there was no significant difference between the total heterograft and Starr-Edwards valve groups in terms of linearized rates of endocarditis (percentage per patient-year). Of the total of 2,184 patients, 51 (2.3%) had prosthetic valve endocarditis. In both the mechanical and tissue valve groups, aortic valve infections were significantly more common than mitral valve involvement.

The increased risk of endocarditis after aortic valve replacement has been corroborated by Sande et al.[30] On the other hand, Magilligan et al.[28] found that mitral valve endocarditis was more common than the aortic variety in patients with heterograft valve endocarditis. Rossiter et al.[29] reported that although the overall incidence of endocarditis was similar in the two valve groups, a higher proportion of patients with infected tissue valves (6/16) sustained early prosthetic valve endocarditis (within 2 weeks after surgery) than did patients with mechanical valves (3/35).

All of these early postoperative heterograft valve infections occurred in aortic valves. Aortocoronary bypass with the saphenous vein was performed more often in combination with tissue valve replacement than with Starr-Edwards valve placement; this procedure could be associated with an increased risk of bacterial contamination from the groin. Analysis of the bypass operation as a separate variable did not explain the higher rate of early prosthetic valve endocarditis in these patients. Magilligan et al.[28] reported that in their series of 373 patients undergoing implantation of heterograft valves, all 11 cases of prosthetic valve endocarditis occurred late postoperatively.

Although there appears to be no difference in the risk of infection between mechanical valves and heterograft valves, heterograft valves, once infected, appear to be more easily sterilized than Starr-Edwards valves and less likely to be associated with the extension of infection past the valve.

CONCLUSIONS AND PRACTICAL RECOMMENDATIONS

The most devastating postoperative infection after cardiac surgery is prosthetic valve endocarditis, usually due to *S. aureus* or *S. epidermidis*. Accordingly, prophylaxis should be directed against these organisms. The ideal regimen is yet to be determined. Short-term perioperative cephalothin administration (8 doses) is as effective as a 4-day or 6-day regimen.

Cefazolin, which is used in many medical centers, appears to be as efficacious as cephalothin; cefazolin, 1 g, should be administered preoperatively and every 8 hours thereafter for 48 hours. There is no evidence that a longer course is required in any subgroup of patients. Newer cephalosporins such as cefoxitin or cefamandole and the "third-generation" cephalosporins have not been demonstrated to be more effective, less costly, or less toxic than cephalothin or cefazolin, and therefore they are not recommended.

Investigational cephalosporins with long half-lives may be useful for single-dose preoperative prophylaxis. This use will require confirmation in controlled clinical trials.

REFERENCES

1. ELLIS LB, HARKEN DE: The clinical results in the first five hundred patients with mitral stenosis undergoing valvuloplasty. Circulation 1955;11:637.

2. KITTLE CF, REED WA: Antibiotics and extracorporeal circulation. J Thorac Cardiovasc Surg 1961;41:34.

3. LORD JW Jr, IMPARATO AM, HACKEL A et al: Endocarditis complicating open-heart surgery. Circulation 1961;23:489.

4. SLONIM R, LITWAK RS, GADBOYS HL et al: Antibiotic prophylaxis of infection complicating open-heart operations. Antimicrob Agents Chemother 1963;3:731.

5. GERACI JE, DALE AJD, McGOON DC: Bacterial endocarditis and endarteritis following cardiac operations. Wis Med J 1963;62:302.

6. HOLSWADE GR, DINEEN P, REDO SF et al: Antibiotic therapy in open-heart operations. Arch Surg 1964;89:970.

7. NELSON RM, JENSON CB, PETERSON CA et al: Effective use of prophylactic antibiotics in open heart surgery. Arch Surg 1965;90:731.

8. REED WA: Antibiotics and cardiac surgery. J Thorac Cardiovasc Surg 1965;50:888.

9. AMOURY RA, BOWMAN FO Jr, MALM JR: Endocarditis associated with intracardiac prostheses. J Thorac Cardiovasc Surg 1966;51:36.

10. STEIN PD, HARKEN DE, DEXTER L: The nature and prevention of prosthetic valve endocarditis. Am Heart J 1966;71:393.

11. FIROR WB: Infection following open-heart surgery, with special reference to the role of prophylactic antibiotics. J Thorac Cardiovasc Surg 1967;53:371.

12. LERNER PI, WEINSTEIN L: Infective endocarditis in the antibiotic era. N Engl J Med 1966;274:199, 259, 323, 388.

13. NEWSOM SWB, LEE WR, REES JR: Fatal fungal infection following open-heart surgery. Br Heart J 1967;29:457.

14. GOODMAN JS, SCHAFFNER W, COLLINS HA et al: Infection after cardiovascular surgery: Clinical study including examination of antimicrobial prophylaxis. N Engl J Med 1968; 278:117.

15. FEKETY FR Jr, CLUFF LE, SABISTON DC Jr et al: A study of antibiotic prophylaxis in cardiac surgery. J Thorac Cardiovasc Surg 1969;57:757.

16. CONTE JE Jr, COHEN SN, ROE BB et al: Antibiotic prophylaxis and cardiac surgery: A prospective double-blind comparison of single-dose versus multiple-dose regimens. Ann Intern Med 1972;76:943.

17. GOLDMANN DA, HOPKINS CC, KARCHMER AW et al: Cephalothin prophylaxis in cardiac valve surgery. J Thorac Cardiovasc Surg 1977;73:470.

18. KINI PM, FERNANDEZ J, CAUSAY RS et al: Double-blind comparison of cefazolin and cephalothin in open-heart surgery. J Thorac Cardiovasc Surg 1978;76:506.

19. MUERS MF, ARNOLD AG, SLEIGHT P: Prophylactic antibiotics for cardiac pacemaker implantation. Br Heart J 1981;46:539.

20. ARCHER GL, TENENBAUM MJ: Antibiotic-resistant *Staphylococcus epidermidis* in patients undergoing cardiac surgery. Antimicrob Agents Chemother 1980;17:269.

21. ARCHER GL, POLK RE, DUMA RJ et al: Comparison of cephalothin and cefamandole prophylaxis during insertion of prosthetic heart valves. Antimicrob Agents Chemother 1978;13:924.

22. WILLIAMS DJ, STEELE TW: Cephalothin prophylaxis assay during cardiopulmonary bypass. J Thorac Cardiovasc Surg 1976;71:207.

23. PIEN FD, MICHAEL NL, MAMIYA R et al: Comparative study of prophylactic antibiotics in cardiac surgery: Clindamycin versus cephalothin. J Thorac Cardiovasc Surg 1979; 77:908.

24. HIRSCHMANN JV, INUI TS: Antimicrobial prophylaxis: A critique of recent trials. Rev Infect Dis 1980;2:1.

25. OYER PE, STINSON EB, GRIEPP RB et al: Valve replacement with the Starr-Edwards and Hancock prostheses: Comparative analysis of late morbidity and mortality. Ann Surg 1977;186:301.

26. YARBOROUGH JW, ROBERTS WC, REIS RL: Structural alterations in tissue cardiac valves implanted in patients and in calves. J Thorac Cardiovasc Surg 1973;65:364.

27. CLARKSON PM, BARRATT-BOYES BG: Bacterial endocarditis following homograft replacement of the aortic valve. Circulation 1970;42:987.

28. MAGILLIGAN DJ Jr, QUINN EL, DAVILA JC: Bacteremia, endocarditis, and the Hancock valve. Ann Thorac Surg 1977;24:508.

29. ROSSITER SJ, STINSON EB, OYER PE et al: Prosthetic valve endocarditis: Comparison of heterograft tissue valves and mechanical valves. J Thorac Cardiovasc Surg 1978; 76:795.

30. SANDE MA, JOHNSON WD Jr, HOOK EW et al: Sustained bacteremia in patients with prosthetic cardiac valves. N Engl J Med 1972;286:1067.

Chapter 5

VASCULAR SURGERY

Issues pertinent to vascular surgery are similar to those in cardiac surgery. The presence or absence of a prosthetic device is crucial, with respect to both likelihood of infection and severity of its consequences. Isolated incisional infection is a nuisance; prosthetic graft infection gravely imperils both life and limb. The site of incision is a major determinant as well, since the groin, lower extremities, abdomen, and chest are at risk of infection in decreasing order of frequency.

CLINICAL STUDIES

As part of a larger study of antibiotic prophylaxis in general surgery, Evans and Pollock[1] included 73 "clean arterial" surgical procedures involving the "lower limbs." The study was prospective and randomized but not blind. Patients were given either three doses of cephaloridine perioperatively or no antibiotic at all. The wound infection rate was significantly reduced. Specific arterial surgical procedures and the use of prostheses were not recorded. One year later, the same group[2] reported the results of a controlled, prospective, randomized but not blind trial of topical cephaloridine prophylaxis in general surgery. Nineteen "clean arterial" procedures were included in this study. Two of 12 (16.7%) wounds in the prophylaxis group and 1 of 4 (25%) wounds in the control group became infected. The difference was not significant.

Subsequently, two well-designed controlled trials, by Kaiser et al.[3] and Pitt et al.,[4] indicated that antibiotic prophylaxis was of value in vascular surgery.

Kaiser et al.[3] prospectively studied 565 patients undergoing abdominal aortic or peripheral vascular surgery. Patients were randomly assigned to receive either placebo or cefazolin before surgery and for 24 hours postoperatively. Individuals were excluded if they were infected or had "wet gangrene" prior to surgery, or if they had a history of serious penicillin or cephalosporin allergy. Wound infections were classified according to depth: class I (superficial), class II (subcutaneous), and class III (graft involvement). No wound infections occurred in 103 patients undergoing carotid or brachial artery surgery irrespective of randomization; thus, midway through the trial, these patients were excluded from the evaluable data.

   Wound infection rates in the remaining 462 who underwent abdominal aortic or lower extremity vascular surgery are summarized in Table 5–1. Of the patients who received placebo, 6.8% became infected ($p < 0.001$). There were no graft infections in the cefazolin group, but there were 4 in the placebo group. Graft infection was associated with serious morbidity (2 amputations) and mortality (2 deaths).

   The highest postoperative infection rate (7.8%) occurred with abdominal aortic resection. Among those patients in this category receiving placebo, the infection rate was 11.8% (6/51), and in those receiving cefazolin it was 2.6% (1/39) ($p < 0.05$). As mentioned previously, brachiocephalic vascular procedures were not associated with postoperative infection. Wound infection developed in 10 of 200 patients (5%) who underwent femoral-lower leg bypass surgery. In this subgroup, the infection rates were 1% (1/105) and 8.7% (9/103), respectively, in those patients receiving cefazolin or placebo ($p < 0.01$).

   Kaiser et al.[3] also noted that the overall wound infection rate was 10.3% in those patients in whom a hexachlorophene-alcohol scrub was used; the rate was reduced to 2.8% if a povidone-iodine scrub was used instead ($p < 0.01$). In patients receiving placebo prophylaxis and a hexachlorophene-alcohol scrub, the postoperative infection rate was high (18%). This was reduced to 0 in patients receiving hexachlorophene-alcohol and cefazolin prophylaxis. Thus, the protective effect of cefazolin prophylaxis was somewhat predictably greatest in the subgroup with the highest infection rate.

   The most common organism isolated from wound infection was *Staphylococcus aureus* (50% of all pathogens). Gram-negative bacilli, alone or in mixed infections, were the second most common

Table 5–1. Wound Infections Among Patients Receiving Cefazolin Prophylaxis or Placebo*

| | Number of Infections | Number of Patients | Percent Infected | Number of Infections by Category | | |
				Class I	Class II	Class III
Prophylaxis						
Cefazolin	2	225	0.9%[†]	0	2	0
Placebo	16	237	6.8%[†]	4	8	4
Total	18	462	3.9%			

*Brachiocephalic procedures are not included.
[†]The difference is significant ($p < 0.001$).
From Kaiser et al,[3] with permission.

Table 5–2. Cephradine Prophylaxis for Vascular Surgery, and Rates of Incisional Infection

		Antibiotic Prophylaxis			
	I No Antibiotic	II Topical Cephradine	III Intravenous Cephradine	IV Topical and Intravenous Cephradine	All Groups
Patient infections					
Infections*/patients	13/53	0/46	0/55	3/51	16/205
Patients infected	24.5%	0†	0	5.9†‡§	7.8%
Incisional infections					
Infections*/incisions	14/62	0/54	0/56	3/59	12/231
Incisions infected	22.6%	0†	0‡	5.1*‡§	7.4%

*Grade II or III groin wound infection.

†$p < 0.01$; no antibiotic vs topical (I vs II or I vs II and IV).

‡$p < 0.01$; no antibiotic vs intravenous (I vs III or I vs III and IV).

§$p < 0.01$; no antibiotic vs topical and intravenous (I vs IV).

From Pitt et al,[4] with permission.

group of organisms. Short-term perioperative prophylaxis, as used in this study, did not favor the development of cefazolin-resistant organisms. Adverse effects (rash and phlebitis) were evaluated as part of the double-blind protocol. The side effects potentially associated with the antibiotic occurred more commonly in the placebo group (4/237) than in the cefazolin group (0/255).

Kaiser et al.[3] concluded that perioperative cefazolin prophylaxis was effective in abdominal and extremity vascular surgery. Infection rates, however, after brachiocephalic vascular procedures are extremely low, and prophylaxis is not warranted in this anatomic site. Finally, the combination of cefazolin and a povidone-iodine scrub was associated with no toxicity, and cefazolin-resistant organisms did not emerge.

Pitt et al.[4] compared topical or systemic cephradine (or both) with no prophylaxis in patients undergoing vascular surgery. The study was prospective, single-blind, and randomized, and included only patients having procedures with groin incisions. Patients were excluded if (1) aortoiliac graft was anticipated, or (2) there was a history of serious penicillin or cephalosporin allergy, or (3) cellulitis or "wet gangrene" of the lower extremity was present at the time of surgery. Patients were randomly allocated to one of four groups: (I) no prophylaxis, (II) incisional cephradine before closure, (III) perioperative intravenous cephradine, and (IV) incisional and intravenous cephradine. All patients received a preoperative scrub with a povidone-iodine solution.

The rate of groin infections was greater in the "no prophylaxis" group (24.5%) than in the topical (0), intravenous (0), or combined topical and intravenous cephradine groups (5.9%) (Table 5–2). Although more graft infections occurred in the "no prophylaxis group" than in the antibiotic groups, these differences did not achieve statistical significance (Table 5–3). As in the study of Kaiser et al., *S. aureus* was the most common cause of wound infection. The remaining organisms isolated were gram-negative rods and enterococci. Sensitivity patterns of these pathogens were not reported by the authors.

Data from the study of Evans and Pollock[1] indicated that parenteral preoperative cephaloridine was of no value in preventing infection after varicose vein surgery. However, the number of patients studied was small. In a larger study, Lord et al.[5] concluded that intraoperative irrigation with cephalothin and kanamycin prevented infection after varicose vein surgery.

Table 5-3. Cephradine Prophylaxis for Vascular Surgery and Rates of Graft Infection (Infections/Patients [%])

| | Antibiotic Prophylaxis | | | | |
	I No Antibiotic	II Topical Cephradine	III Intravenous Cephradine	IV Topical and Intravenous Cephradine	All Groups
Patient infections					
Synthetic graft present*	3[†]/13 (23.1)	0/10 (0)	0/14 (0)	1[†]/15 (6.7)	4/52 (7.7)
No synthetic graft	10/40 (25.0)	0/36 (0)	0/41 (0)	2/36 (5.6)	12/153 (7.8)
Incisional infections					
Synthetic graft present*	3/18 (16.7)	0/16 (0)	0/17 (0)	1/25 (4.0)	4/76 (5.2)
No synthetic graft	11/44 (25.0)	0/38 (0)	0/39 (0)	2/34 (5.9)	13/135 (8.4)

*Dacron—44 patients, 67 incisions; Gortex—8 patients, 9 incisions.
[†] No loss of limb or life upon follow-up of 10, 28, 29, and 35 months.
From Pitt et al.,[4] with permission.

PHARMACOLOGIC CONSIDERATIONS

Antibiotic Selection

The investigators in the controlled trials already discussed used prophylaxis with a cephalosporin, a reasonable choice when one considers the cause of postoperative infection in this group of patients. May et al.[6] compared cephalothin with oxacillin prophylaxis in vascular surgery. They noted no significant differences when the groups were analyzed for rates of wound, graft, urinary, or pulmonary infection.

Route of Administration

Considerable experimental and clinical data suggest that topically applied antibiotics may provide protection against postoperative wound infection.[5,7–9] Lord et al.,[5] in a retrospective study of patients undergoing vascular procedures, reported only 1 wound infection among 434 patients (0.23%) given topical cephalothin and kanamycin prophylaxis; this incidence compared favorably with a 1.5% incidence of infection among 400 patients operated on previously with no antibiotic prophylaxis. Lord et al. also conducted a prospective, randomized, and blind study of topical antibiotics in 200 patients undergoing operations for varicose veins. No grade II wound infections were noted in either the antibiotic or placebo group, although minor skin changes did occur less frequently among those patients whose incisions were irrigated with an antibiotic solution.

In contrast, Evans and Pollock[2,10] reported rates of groin wound infection greater than 25% despite the use of topical antibiotics.

More recently, Pitt et al.[4] showed that topical prophylaxis is as effective as systemic prophylaxis and that the combination has no advantage over either route alone. Suppression of bacteremia appears to be unimportant, since the vast majority of graft infections result from infection of the groin incision.

EXPERIMENTAL ASPECTS

Investigators[11] tested collagen as a carrier for various substances, including antibiotics. Collagen-bonding prevents immediate washout and could conceivably maintain antibacterial activity on the bonded surface for prolonged periods. Moore et al.[12] suggested that it would be important to maintain antibiotic activity at the graft site for approximately 3 weeks after implantation. From a clinical standpoint, this would take the patient beyond the risk of perioperative bacterial exposure. Additional requirements for an antibiotic release system are that the system provide tight bonding to the fabric, that it be safe, and that it be nonfibrogenic. Such a system might be considerably more effective than passive antibiotic soaking of a prosthesis.[13,14]

PRACTICAL SURGICAL RECOMMENDATIONS

Clinical trials[3,4] indicated that cephalosporin prophylaxis is useful in vascular surgery. One[4] of two well-designed studies reported that intraoperative topical prophylaxis was as good as perioperative parenteral prophylaxis. The value of prophylaxis in varicose vein surgery is unclear and requires further study.

The primary purpose of antibiotic prophylaxis in vascular surgery is the prevention of graft infection. When choosing a prophylactic antibiotic for vascular surgery, one should consider two important factors: The first is the spectrum of organisms that one is likely to encounter, including staphylococci, Enterobacteriaceae, and other gram-negative bacteria.[6] Second, the route of administration and timing are important; high serum concentrations of antibiotic should be present just before and during surgery. Prophylaxis should be short to avoid toxicity and superinfection by resistant strains and to reduce costs.[15,16] Cephalosporins, which have been widely studied, are suitable for prophylaxis by reason of their spectrum of activity, pharmacokinetics, and comparative safety.

Postoperative wound infection rates are highest for abdominal or lower extremity vascular procedures,[17] and prophylaxis is justified in these cases. Cefazolin, 1 g, should be given intramuscularly or intravenously, 1 to 2 hours preoperatively and every 8 hours thereafter for 24 hours.

The rates of wound infection after brachiocephalic and carotid vascular procedures are extremely low, and therefore prophylaxis is not indicated in these cases.

REFERENCES

1. EVANS C, POLLOCK AV: The reduction of surgical wound infections by prophylactic parenteral cephaloridine. Br J Surg 1973;60:434.
2. EVANS C, POLLOCK AV, ROSENBERG IL: The reduction of surgical wound infections by topical cephaloridine: A controlled clinical trial. Br J Surg 1974;61:133.
3. KAISER AB, CLAYSON KR, MULHERIN JL Jr et al: Antibiotic prophylaxis in vascular surgery. Ann Surg 1978;188:283.
4. PITT HA, POSTIER RG, MacGOWAN WAL et al: Prophylactic antibiotics in vascular surgery. Ann Surg 1980;192:356.
5. LORD JW Jr, ROSSI G, DALIANA M: Intraoperative antibiotic wound lavage: An attempt to eliminate postoperative infection in arterial and clean general surgical procedures. Ann Surg 1977;185:634.
6. MAY ARL, DARLING RC, BREWSTER DC et al: A comparison of the use of cephalothin and oxacillin in vascular surgery. Arch Surg 1980;115:56.
7. HALASZ NA: Wound infection and topical antibiotics: The surgeon's dilemma. Arch Surg 1977;112:1240.
8. ALEXANDER JW, ALEXANDER NS: The influence of route of administration on wound fluid concentration of prophylactic antibiotics. J Trauma 1976;16:488.
9. SCHERR DD, DODD TA: Brief exposure of bacteria to topical antibiotics. Surg Gynecol Obstet 1973;137:87.
10. POLLOCK AV, EVANS C: The prophylaxis of surgical wound sepsis with cephaloridine: Experiences in 2491 general surgical operations and reporting a controlled clinical trial against framycetin. J Antimicrob Chemother 1975;1,Suppl 3:71.
11. KRAJICEK M, DVORAK J, CHVAPIL M: Infection-resistant synthetic vascular substitutes. J Cardiovasc Surg 1969;10:453.
12. MOORE WS, CHVAPIL M, SEIFFERT G et al: Development of an infection-resistant vascular prosthesis. Arch Surg 1981;116:1403.

13. RICHARDSON RL Jr, PATE JW, WOLF RY et al: The outcome of anti-
    biotic-soaked arterial grafts in guinea pig wounds
    contaminated with *E. coli* or *S. aureus*. J Thorac Cardiovasc
    Surg 1970;59:635.
14. BAKER WH, BODENSTEINER JA: The administration of antibiotics
    in vascular reconstructive surgery. J Thorac Cardiovasc
    Surg 1972;64:301.
15. BURKE JF: Preoperative antibiotics. Surg Clin North Am
    1963;43:665.
16. LINTON RR: The prophylactic use of the antibiotics in clean
    surgery. Surg Gynecol Obstet 1961;112:218 (Editorial).
17. MALONE JM, MOORE WS, CAMPAGNA G et al: Bacteremic infect-
    ability of vascular grafts: The influence of pseudointimal
    integrity and duration of graft function. Surgery 1975;
    78:211.

Chapter *6*

ORTHOPEDIC SURGERY

Many clinicians believe that because the infection rate associated with clean surgery is so low, the costs and adverse effects of antibiotic prophylaxis exceed the benefits in most instances. This is true except in procedures such as artificial joint implantation and hip arthroplasty, in which an infection would likely result in a catastrophic outcome. Few orthopedic surgical cases fall into the clean-contaminated category, which, in most surgical specialties, constitutes the principal group of patients to receive and benefit from antibiotic prophylaxis. Contaminated or dirty operations are common in orthopedic surgical procedures for traumatic injuries. In these categories, bacteria are already present in the operative site; the use of antimicrobial agents therefore represents therapy rather than prophylaxis.

Although local wound irrigation with bacitracin, neomycin, or polymyxin used alone or in combination is commonplace in orthopedic surgery, no data exist to support the use of routine antibiotic irrigations. In addition, no beneficial effect has been demonstrated in elective procedures with the routine attempt to purify the air in the operating room with ultraviolet light.

Total joint replacement is a clean surgical procedure. The prime considerations in the prevention of infection are careful surgical asepsis and technique and gentle handling of tissues. Additional measures have been used to reduce the incidence of postoperative infection and the significant morbidity and economic costs associated with it.

Charnley[1,2] advocated reduction of exogenous operative wound contamination by unidirectional air flow, ultrafiltered air, rapid air changes, ultrafine fabrics for clothing and drapes, and special air exhaust systems. Other investigators[3-5] favor ultraviolet light in the operating room to reduce contamination and the incidence of postoperative wound infection. The effectiveness of these measures remains controversial.[6] The most widely used means of reducing the incidence of infection after total hip replacement is preoperative, intraoperative, and early postoperative antibiotic prophylaxis. This method is based on evidence indicating that most operative wound infections are endogenous rather than exogenous.

CLINICAL STUDIES

As discussed in Chapter 1, one of the earliest attempts to use antibiotics prophylactically was in orthopedic trauma.[7] Antibiotic prophylaxis in "clean" orthopedic surgery has been reported from a number of centers. These studies were largely retrospective and therefore seldom controlled and not randomized. The investigators[8-17] used nonstandard antibiotic regimens, intermixed patients in different surgical categories, or included patients for whom prophylaxis was provided only postoperatively.

Pavel et al.[18] studied the effect of cephaloridine prophylaxis during 1,591 "clean" orthopedic procedures. The trial was prospective and placebo-controlled, and used a standard regimen. Cephaloridine was given preoperatively and intraoperatively. The infection rates in 887 patients who received prophylaxis and in 704 patients who received placebo were 2.8% and 5%, respectively. This difference was statistically significant, and the authors therefore concluded that antibiotic prophylaxis for clean orthopedic surgery was effective in reducing postoperative infection. No data as to bacteriologic effects or wound outcome were included in this study.

Erickson et al.[19] evaluated parenteral cloxacillin prophylaxis in a double-blind prospective study of patients who underwent Charnley total hip implants, Moore prosthesis arthroplasty, or Thornton nail repair of femoral fractures. Infection was significantly reduced only in the group having Charnley total hip implants (Table 6–1). All of these infections were detected within 2 weeks after

Table 6–1. Incidence of Infection in Cloxacillin and Placebo Groups

	Cloxacillin			Placebo	
	Total	Infected	Not Infected	Infected	Not Infected
Charnley total hip	118	0	60	10 (17%)	48 ($p < 0.001$)
Moore prosthesis	14	0	5	1	8 ($p < 0.05$)
Thornton nail	39	0	18	1	20 ($p < 0.05$)

From Ericson et al.,[19] with permission.

surgery. Ten of the 12 infections were due to *Staphylococcus aureus;* one was mixed infection with *Proteus mirabilis.* One patient was infected with *Staphylococcus epidermidis* and one had a mixed *Pseudomonas aeruginosa* and *Klebsiella* infection. Follow-up analysis[20] by the same group of investigators revealed an excessive incidence of late infection in the group receiving placebo (Table 6–2). The authors[20] concluded that cloxacillin prophylaxis was effective in preventing early and late postoperative infection associated with total hip replacement.

Visuri et al.[21] compared dicloxacillin and ampicillin, and Wilson[22] studied oxacillin prophylaxis for patients having total hip replacements. Both groups of investigators concluded that anti-staphylococcal prophylaxis was of value in total hip replacement (THR); however, these were not randomized, prospective studies.

Pollard et al.[23] studied 297 patients undergoing total hip replacement. In a prospective, randomized (but not blind) trial, one group received cephaloridine, 1 g intraoperatively, followed by 1 g at 6 and 12 hours postoperatively, and the other group received flucloxacillin, 500 mg intravenously during the operation and then every 6 hours for 14 days. Overall deep (1.3%) and superficial (1.65%) infection rates were low, and there were no significant differences between the two groups. Of 9 infections, 4 were due to unspeciated gram-negative rods, 2 to *S. aureus,* and 1 each to *S. epidermidis, Streptococcus faecalis,* and anaerobic diphtheroids. Because of the small number of infections, selection of resistant organisms could not be attributed to either regimen.

Schulitz et al.[24] studied 259 patients undergoing total hip replacement. The trial was prospective and randomized, and included a control group that received no prophylaxis. The investigators compared two 600-mg doses of lincomycin given 1 and 6 hours postoperatively, again on the first postoperative day, followed by 1 g orally three times a day from the third to the tenth postoperative day. Sixty-five of the 259 patients were excluded from the study; 194 studies were analyzed (Table 6–3). The rates for all infections and deep infection, analyzed separately, were significantly lower in the antibiotic group. The most common infective organism was *S. aureus.* Others included *E. coli,* "enterococcus," *Klebsiella, Pseudomonas,* and *Achromobacter.* The authors concluded that lincomycin prophylaxis reduced the deep infection rate associated with total hip replacement from approximately 9% to 1%.

The only double-blind randomized trial of antibiotic prophylaxis for total hip replacement was recently reported by Hill et

Table 6–2. Incidence of Late Hip Infection

		Cloxacillin		Placebo		
	Total	Not Infected	Infected	Not Infected	Infected	
1-2½ years postoperatively	118	60	0	51	7	(p < 0.05)*
5-6½ years postoperatively	118	58	2	44	14	(p < 0.01)*

*Chi-square with Yates correction.
Modified from data of Carlsson et al.,[20] with permission.

Table 6–3. Reduction in Infection Rates Associated with Total Hip Replacement by Lincomycin Prophylaxis

	All Infections		Deep Infections		
	Yes (%)	No (%)	Yes (%)	No (%)	Total Patients
Lincomycin group	3 (2.9)	102 (97)	1 (0.9)	104 (99)	105
Control group	10 (11.2)*	79 (77.4)	8 (9.9)†	81 (91)	89

*$0.025 < p < 0.05$.
†$0.01 < p < 0.025$.
Modified from data of Schulitz et al.,[24] with permission.

al.[25] In a multicenter trial involving 9 hospitals and 2,097 patients, they compared cefazolin prophylaxis, 1 g every 6 hours for 6 days, with placebo. Postoperative hip infection was reduced from 3.3% in the placebo group to 0.9% in the cefazolin group. The difference was highly significant ($p < 0.001$).

In addition, the authors[25] presented data indicating that infection rates in other sites (urinary, pulmonary, gastrointestinal) were not increased by the use of cefazolin prophylaxis. Moreover, patients with "risk factors" (for example, diabetes, obesity, alcoholism) did not have higher infection rates than patients without "risk factors." Positive intraoperative specimen cultures and drain cultures were significantly more common in patients suffering postoperative hip infection than in those who did not. There was no relation between urinary tract infection within 2 weeks after surgery and postoperative hip infection. The results of bacteriologic studies were not included in this report.

MICROBIOLOGIC CONSIDERATIONS

The main emphasis in prophylaxis for orthopedic surgical cases has been coverage of gram-positive organisms, especially *S. aureus* and, less often, *S. epidermidis*. However, recent studies have suggested an evolution toward gram-negative organisms as causative agents in deep and superficial wound infections after orthopedic surgical procedures.

Wilson et al.[26] reported a change in bacterial isolates after joint replacement, from a ratio of 81% gram-positive and 19% gram-negative organisms in 1968 to a 64%-70% gram-positive and a 27%-36% gram-negative ratio in the years 1970 to 1975. During these 6 years, the bacterial isolates showed a preponderance of staphylococcal organisms (31% *S. aureus,* 20% *S. epidermidis*), with enterococcus 10%, *Proteus* sp. 8.3%, *E. coli* 6.8%, *Klebsiella* sp. 6.8%, *Pseudomonas* sp. 6.8%, and *Enterobacter* sp. 2.6%. Similarly, Andrews et al.[27] reported that 36% of isolates from total hip replacement infection were gram-negative organisms. Irvine et al.[28] have reported the spread of gram-negative urinary tract infections to total joint implants. Fitzgerald et al.[29] reported that 73% of their isolates from deep infection after total hip arthroplasty were gram-positive and 27% were gram-negative. Twenty-five of their 49 isolates were staphylococcal (*S. aureus* in 10, *S. epidermidis* in 8, and the anaerobe *Peptococcus* in 7). With increasing physician awareness and improved culturing techniques, anaerobic organisms are being increasingly identified as causative agents in orthopedic infections. Fitzgerald et al. reported that anaerobic bacteria recovered from infected hip cases constituted 22% of all bacterial isolates. The true role of anaerobes in orthopedic infections will be understood only when appropriate anaerobic culture techniques are widely used in orthopedic infections. It seems appropriate that antimicrobal prophylaxis be aimed at the commonly identified pathogens. Thus, in orthopedic surgery an agent should be administered that is primarily effective against penicillin-resistant strains of *S. aureus, S. epidermidis,* and gram-negative enteric bacteria such as *E. coli, Klebsiella,* and *Proteus.*

PHARMACOLOGIC CONSIDERATIONS

Duration of Prophylaxis

Pollard et al.[23] compared a three-dose course of cephaloridine with flucloxacillin given for 14 days after total hip replacement in 290 patients. Deep infection occurred in only 4 patients, 2 in each group. Hill et al.[25] compared a 5-day regimen of cefazolin with placebo and demonstrated that prophylaxis reduced the infection rate from 3.3% to 0.9%. Thus, a 14-day course of antibiotic prophylaxis is not necessary, and a 5-day regimen appears to yield no better results than a three-dose regimen.

Drug Selection

Antibiotics that are used prophylactically have different chemical, pharmacokinetic, and antibacterial properties. In addition, there is considerable between-subject and intraindividual variation in the antibiotic concentrations in different parts of the bone. Possible causes include differences in distribution and penetration of antibiotics between adjacent parts of the same bone fragment, the avidity with which the antibiotic binds to tissue proteins within bone, and the ratio between the amount of protein-free antibiotic in the intravascular haversian canal systems of bone and that which reaches extravascular (for example, cortical) bone.[30] Moreover, the wound in bone differs from that in soft tissue; in bone the wound invariably contains a large hematoma. The avascularity of the hematoma protects any bacterial inoculum from circulating antibacterial agents and allows the hematoma to act as a culture medium for bacterial growth.

Prophylactic antimicrobial therapy to prevent infection during total joint arthroplasty has resulted in numerous in vivo studies in an attempt to delineate the ability of various antimicrobials to penetrate bone. Comparison[31] of the results of in vivo studies of the concentrations of antimicrobials in bone is difficult. Various surgical procedures are used to obtain osseous specimens. Schurman et al.[32] maintained that specimens obtained during total knee arthroplasty, which is performed under a tourniquet, permitted an accurate reflection of the osseous drug concentration. In contrast, Cunha et al.[33] demonstrated at least a 40% reduction of the osseous drug concentration when a tourniquet was used.

Many authors fail to identify the underlying pathologic process for which reconstruction was performed. Specimens obtained from the necrotic region of an osteonecrotic femoral head or the sclerotic region of the osteoarthritic femoral head would reflect the altered vascular supply and, therefore, an osseous drug concentration that is not representative. The time when the osseous specimen is obtained after the antimicrobial injection is also important if proper comparisons are to be made.

Schurman et al.[34] reported that the bone concentration of cefamandole, a "second-generation" cephalosporin, was higher by a factor of 3 than that of cephalothin. Of additional interest was that the concentrations of the same antibiotic at the hip and knee were not significantly different even though a tourniquet was used for the knee replacement procedures. Patel et al.[35] found measurable amounts of cephalothin in at least one bone specimen of all patients.

Kopta and Lesken[36] demonstrated that bone concentrations of cefazolin in rabbits remained high even after serum levels had decreased. The study of Pitkin et al.[37] corroborated this finding.

Parsons,[38] who reviewed the subject of antibiotics in bone, concluded that cefazolin was the antibiotic of choice for prophylactic use in patients undergoing total hip replacement. He demonstrated cefazolin bone concentrations well above the minimal bactericidal concentrations for *S. aureus* and those gram-negative organisms causing postoperative prosthetic infections.

Cefotaxime, a "third-generation" semisynthetic cephalosporin with a high degree of stability to β-lactamases from gram-negative bacteria, produced bone levels that were satisfactory when a dosage of 2 g intramuscularly every 8 hours was used.[39] Cefonicid, an investigational cephalosporin, achieved bone levels of 14 μg per gram of crushed bone after a single dose of 1 g intramuscularly (personal communication from C. Nightingale, 1982). Such high bone concentrations probably result from the high serum concentrations ($>$ 100 μg/ml) achievable with a single 1-g intramuscular dose.

Patel et al.[35] reported that induced hypotension during total hip replacement might result in reduced antibiotic levels in bone. When pentolinium was used to induce hypotension, bone concentrations of cephalothin were lower; this was not true for trimethophan-induced hypotension. The authors suggested that although both agents are ganglionic-blockers, trimethophan also has a direct vasodilating effect on peripheral blood vessels, resulting in improved bone perfusion and higher antibiotic bone concentrations.[35]

Fitzgerald et al.[31] studied the penetration of methicillin, oxacillin, and cephalothin into cortical bone and synovial tissues. Samples were obtained 1 hour after intravenous administration of antibiotic. Cephalothin usually reached concentrations in cortical bone that were inhibitory for staphylococci. The high protein-binding of oxacillin did not alter its penetration into osseous or synovial tissues, and there were no significant differences in the concentrations of methicillin and oxacillin in these tissues.

Using antibiotics in cement as a prophylactic measure was advocated in 1970 by Buchholz and Engelbrecht.[40] Moore[41] addressed the efficacy and advisability of this practice. Concerns have been raised over such factors as antibiotic choice, effective local tissue antibiotic concentration over time, toxic or allergic reactions, and emergence of resistant organisms. The effect of antibiotic additives on the mechanical integrity of the cement must also be considered, especially in the light of observations by Markhoff and Amstutz[42] suggesting that cement failure is a precursor of gross loosening and femoral stem failure.

Wahlig and Dingeldein[43] studied release kinetics of several antibiotics from different bone cements in animals and humans. Antibiotics administered with bone cements are known to leach out of the hardened plastic material by diffusion. The amount measurable in vitro has been found to be proportional to the surface area of the cement. These studies have demonstrated that not every bone cement or antibiotic is suitable for use in an antibiotic bone cement mixture for all arthroplasty. Among 12 different antibiotics, only gentamicin and lincomycin-clindamycin were found to be released in amounts that seemed to be sufficient, if concentrations were correlated with the antibacterial activity of the compounds.

The effect of antibiotics on the mechanical properties of polymethylmethacrylate has been reported by several investigators. No significant differences have been reported in compressive and tensile strengths with 5% gentamicin, oxacillin, and cefazolin in powder form.[44] It has, however, been demonstrated that compressive and tensile strengths are decreased by 2 g, 4 g, and 8 g of gentamicin or cephalothin in Simplex P.

ORTHOPEDIC TRAUMA

Clinical Studies and Microbiologic Considerations

In 1973, Boyd et al.[45] reported on the use of antibiotic prophylaxis in 417 patients undergoing surgery for hip fracture. The study was prospective, double-blind, and randomized; it compared nafcillin, 0.5 g intravenously before and during operation, followed by 0.5 g intravenously every 6 hours for 48 hours; placebo was given in the same manner. The authors reported a decrease in wound infection rate from 4.8% (7 of 145 patients) in the placebo group to 0.7% (1 of 135 patients) in the nafcillin group. However, analysis of these data is difficult because of the large number of exclusions from the study (19%). One reviewer[46] believed that the report was therefore unevaluable.

In this series, all infections in the nafcillin group were due to *S. aureus* except two (one *E. coli* and one mixed *E. coli* and *Proteus* sp.). In the placebo group a greater variety of organisms was encountered: *S. aureus, Staphylococcus albus, P. mirabilis,* anaerobic diphtheroids, *E. coli,* β-hemolytic streptococci and mixed *Klebsiella,* diphtheroids, and nonhemolytic streptococci. The authors[46] concluded that there was no significant correlation among microbiologic data, type of fracture, and orthopedic device, and further that "there was nothing to suggest that the type and sensitivity of the bacteria were influenced by the antibiotics given prophylactically."

The role of short-term cephalosporin prophylaxis in 140 patients undergoing surgery for trochanteric fracture in Sweden was evaluated by Tengve and Kjellander.[47] The prophylaxis group received intravenous cephalothin 2 g preoperatively and intraoperatively, followed by 2 g intravenously every 6 hours or 1 g of cephalexin every 6 hours for a total of 48 hours. The control group received no antibiotics. The study was not blind, and placebo was not used. Infection occurred in 1 out of 56 patients (1.8%) who received prophylaxis, and in 12 out of 71 (16.9%) in the control group. These infection rates are remarkably similar to those reported by Boyd et al.[45] The wound infection in the one patient who received prophylaxis was due to unspeciated "enterococcus." In the control group infection was due to *S. aureus*, "enterococcus," "anaerobic streptococci," and *"Klebsiella."* The authors concluded that short-term prophylaxis was of value in this type of surgery.

A larger double-blind prospective study performed by Burnett et al.[48] confirmed this observation. Three hundred seven patients undergoing surgery for proximal femoral fractures were studied. The prophylaxis group received, before, during, and after operation, cephalothin, 1 g every 4 hours, and for 72 hours postoperatively. The control group received placebo on the same schedule. Six major postoperative hip infections (4.7%) occurred in the placebo group and one (0.7%) in the cephalothin group. *S. aureus* sensitive to cephalothin was isolated from the wounds of all 6 patients in the placebo group. One of the 6 also had a *E. coli* and α-hemolytic streptococcus and another, group A streptococcus isolated from the wound in addition to the *S. aureus*.

The infection in the patient in the cephalothin group was mixed and contained "alpha-streptococcus" and "coagulase-negative staphylococcus" sensitive to cephalothin, and *"Pseudomonas"* and *"Enterobacter"* resistant to cephalothin.

Moreover, these authors[48] believed that cephalothin prophylaxis may have favored the development of resistant organisms at other sites. Of 32 organisms isolated from other sites in placebo group patients, 7 (22%) were resistant to cephalothin. Of 24 organisms isolated from the cephalothin group patients, 10 (42%) were resistant to cephalothin. This difference, however, did not achieve statistical significance ($p = 0.097$).

There were no major complications of antibiotic prophylaxis. Phlebitis developed in 7 patients in the cephalothin group and 2 in the placebo group; 2 patients in the cephalothin group had fever not attributable to any other source.

The authors[48] concluded that cephalothin prophylaxis significantly decreased the rate of wound infection associated with surgery for hip fracture but noted a disturbing trend toward the development of resistant organisms in the prophylaxis group.

There have been no prospective blind trials of antibiotic prophylaxis in the management of open fractures. Routine use of early antibiotic administration for war wounds did not appear to prevent infection[49]; others also advised against the use of prophylaxis in civilian orthopedic trauma.[50,51]

These studies, however, examined the use of penicillin and streptomycin prophylaxis, which would be expected to be ineffective against most infections caused by *S. aureus*. Patzakis et al.[52] studied 310 patients with open fractures in a prospective randomized trial that was not blind. Group I received no prophylaxis, group II received penicillin and streptomycin for 10 to 14 days, and group III received cephalothin intravenously, 100 mg/kg in four divided doses for 10 to 14 days. There were 11 infections in 79 group I patients (13.9%), 9 infections in 92 group II patients (9.8%), and 2 infections in 84 group III patients (2.4%). The difference between the cephalothin group (group III) and the other two groups was statistically significant ($p < 0.05$).

The most common organism isolated from infections in groups I and II was *S. aureus*; in group III, 2 patients were infected with "mixed gram negatives."

Six patients had adverse antibiotic reactions, 5 in group III and 1 in group II. None of these was judged to be serious.

The authors[52] concluded that the term "prophylaxis" was inappropriate in this setting because intraoperative cultures were positive in 165 of 255 wounds (64.7%). Thus, antibiotic administration in this situation should be regarded as early therapy rather than prophylaxis.

PRACTICAL RECOMMENDATIONS

1. Systemic prophylaxis is justified for patients in whom foreign material (metal or bone grafts) is to be implanted on an elective basis. The current drug of choice is cefazolin

perioperatively, 1 g every 8 hours, although some surgeons use more specific antistaphylococcal agents.

2. Systemic prophylaxis is not warranted in elective orthopedic operations in which implants are not used.

3. Systemic antibiotics are an important adjunct to primary care of the wound, which consists mainly of débridement, achievement of hemostasis, and irrigation, in patients with open or compound fractures. Cefazolin, 1 g every 8 hours, should be administered intravenously or intramuscularly as soon as possible after the injury and should be continued for 7 to 10 days. This use of antibiotics should be regarded as therapeutic rather than prophylactic.

REFERENCES

1. CHARNLEY J: A clean air operating enclosure. Br J Surg 1964;51:202.
2. CHARNLEY J: Postoperative infection after total hip replacement with special reference to air contamination in the operating room. Clin Orthop 1972;87:167.
3. NATIONAL ACADEMY OF SCIENCES–NATIONAL RESEARCH COUNCIL: Postoperative wound infections: The influence of ultraviolet irradiation of the operating room and of various other factors. Report of an Ad Hoc Committee of the Committee on Trauma. Ann Surg 1964;160(Suppl):1.
4. HART D, POSTLETHWAIT RW, BROWN IW Jr et al: Postoperative wound infections: A further report on ultraviolet irradiation with comments on the recent (1964) National Research Council Cooperative Study Report. Ann Surg 1968;167:728.
5. WRIGHT RL, BURKE JF: Effect of ultraviolet radiation on postoperative sepsis. J Neurosurg 1969;31:533.
6. HOWARD RJ: The environment. *In:* Polk HC Jr (ed): Infection and the Surgical Patient. Edinburgh: Churchill Livingstone, 1982;30-41.
7. JENSEN NK, JOHNSRUD LW, NELSON MC: The local implantation of sulfanilamide in compound fractures. Surgery 1939;6:1.

8. TACHDJIAN MO, COMPERE EL: Postoperative wound infections in orthopedic surgery. J Int Coll Surg 1957;28:797.

9. OLIX ML, KLUG TJ, COLEMAN CR et al: Prophylactic penicillin and streptomycin in elective operations on bones, joints and tendons. Surg Forum 1960;10:818.

10. MAGUIRE WB: The use of antibiotics, locally and systemically, in orthopaedic surgery. Med J Aust 1964;2:412.

11. SCHONHOLTZ GJ, BORGIA CA, BLAIR JD: Wound sepsis in orthopaedic surgery. J Bone Joint Surg 1962;44-A:1548.

12. STEVENS DB: Postoperative orthopaedic infections. J Bone Joint Surg 1964;46-A:96.

13. PROTHERO SR, PARKES JC, STINCHFIELD FE: Complications after low-back fusion in 1000 patients. J Bone Joint Surg 1966;48-A:57.

14. DERIAN PS, GREEN BM: Postoperative wound infections: 5-year review of 1163 consecutive operative orthopedic patients. Am Surg 1966;32:388.

15. FOGELBERG EV, ZITZMANN EK, STINCHFIELD FE: Prophylactic penicillin in orthopaedic surgery. J Bone Joint Surg 1970;52-A:95.

16. HORWITZ NH, CURTIN JA: Prophylactic antibiotics and wound infections following laminectomy for lumbar disc herniation. J Neurosurg 1975;43:727.

17. MILLER WE, COUNTS GW: Orthopedic infections: A prospective study of 378 clean procedures. South Med J 1975;68:386.

18. PAVEL A, SMITH RL, BALLARD A et al: Prophylactic antibiotics in clean orthopaedic surgery. J Bone Joint Surg 1974;56-A:777.

19. ERICSON C, LIDGREN L, LINDBERG L: Cloxacillin in the prophylaxis of postoperative infections of the hip. J Bone Joint Surg 1973;55-A:808.

20. CARLSSON AS, LIDGREN L, LINDBERG L: Prophylactic antibiotics against early and late deep infections after total hip replacements. Acta Orthop Scand 1977;48:405.

21. VISURI T, ANTILA P, LAURENT LE: A comparison of dicloxacillin and ampicillin in the antibiotic prophylaxis of total hip replacement. Ann Chir Gynaecol 1976;65:58.

22. WILSON PD Jr: Joint replacement. South Med J 1977;70,Suppl 1:55.

23. POLLARD JP, HUGHES SPF, SCOTT JE et al: Antibiotic prophylaxis in total hip replacement. Br Med J 1979;1:707.

24. SCHULITZ KP, WINKELMANN W, SCHOENING B: The prophylactic use of antibiotics in alloarthroplasty of the hip joint for cox- arthrosis: A randomized study. Arch Orthop Trauma Surg 1980;96:79.

25. HILL C, MAZAS F, FLAMANT R et al: Prophylactic cefazolin versus placebo in total hip replacement. Lancet 1981;1:795.

26. WILSON PD Jr, SALVATI EA, BLUMENFELD EL: The problem of infec- tion in total prosthetic arthroplasty of the hip. Surg Clin North Am 1975;55:1431.

27. ANDREWS HJ, ARDEN GP, HART GM et al: Deep infection after total hip replacement. J Bone Joint Surg 1981;63:53.

28. IRVINE R, JOHNSON BL Jr, AMSTUTZ HC: The relationship of geni- tourinary tract procedures and deep sepsis after total hip replacements. Surg Gynecol Obstet 1974;139:701.

29. FITZGERALD RH Jr, PETERSON LF, WASHINGTON JA II et al: Bacterial colonization of wound and sepsis in total hip arthroplasty. J Bone Joint Surg 1973;55-A:1242.

30. PARSONS RL, BEAVIS JP, LAURENCE M et al: Plasma, bone, hip cap- sule and drain fluid concentrations of ampicillin and flu- cloxacillin during total hip replacement after intravenous bolus injection of magnapen. Br J Clin Pharmacol 1978; 6:135.

31. FITZGERALD RH Jr, KELLY PJ, SNYDER RJ et al: Penetration of methi- cillin, oxacillin, and cephalothin into bone and synovial tissues. Antimicrob Agents Chemother 1978;14:723.

32. SCHURMAN DJ et al: Transactions, 23rd Annual Meeting of Orthopedic Research Society; 1977:30.

33. CUNHA BA, GOSSLING HR, NIGHTINGALE CH et al: Penetration of cefazolin and cephradine into bone in patients undergoing total knee arthroplasty. 17th Interscience Conference on Antimicrobial Agents and Chemotherapy, 1977 (Ab- stract 351).

34. SCHURMAN DJ, HIRSHMAN HP, BURTON DS: Cephalothin and cefamandole penetration into bone, synovial fluid and wound drainage fluid. J Bone Joint Surg 1980;62-A:981.

35. PATEL BD et al: The effect of hypotensive anesthesia on cephalo- thin concentrations in bone and muscle of patients under- going total hip replacement. J Bone Joint Surg 1979; 61-A:531.

36. KOPTA JA, LESKEN P: Presentation to Association of Bone and Joint Surgeons, 1975.

37. PITKIN DH, SACHS C, ZAJAC I et al: Distribution of sodium cefazolin in serum, muscle, bone marrow, and bone of normal rab- bits. Antimicrob Agents Chemother 1977;11:760.

38. PARSONS RL: Antibiotics in bone. J Antimicrob Chemother 1976;2:228.

39. KOSMIDIS J, STATHAKIS C, MANTOPOULOS K et al: Clinical pharmacology of cefotaxime including penetration into bile, sputum, bone and cerebrospinal fluid. J Antimicrob Chemother 1980;6,Suppl A:147.

40. BUCHHOLZ HW, ENGELBRECHT H: Uber die Depotwirkung einiger Antibiotica bei Vermischung mit dem Kunstharz Palacos. Chirurg 1970;41:511.

41. MOORE B: Antibiotics in cement. J Bone Joint Surg 1977; 59:139.

42. MARKOLF KL, AMSTUTZ HC: A comparative experimental study of stresses in femoral total hip replacement components: The effect of prostheses orientation and acrylic fixation. J Biomech 1976;9:73.

43. WAHLIG H, DINGELDEIN E: Antibiotics and bone cements. Acta Orthop Scand 1980;51:49.

44. MARKS KE, NELSON CL, LAUTENSCHLAGER EP: Antibiotic-impregnated acrylic bone cement. J Bone Joint Surg 1976;58-A:358.

45. BOYD RJ, BURKE JF, COLTON T: A double-blind clinical trial of prophylactic antibiotics in hip fractures. J Bone Joint Surg 1973;55-A:1251.

46. CHODAK GW, PLAUT ME: Use of systemic antibiotics for prophylaxis in surgery. Arch Surg 1977;112:326.

47. TENGVE B, KJELLANDER J: Antibiotic prophylaxis in operations on trochanteric femoral fractures. J Bone Joint Surg 1978;60-A:97.

48. BURNETT JW, GUSTILO RB, WILLIAMS DN et al: Prophylactic antibiotics in hip fractures: A double-blind, prospective study. J Bone Joint Surg 1980;62-A:457.

49. KLEIN RS, BERGER SA, YEKUTIEL P: Wound infection during the Yom Kippur War: Observations concerning antibiotic prophylaxis and therapy. Ann Surg 1975;182:15.

50. COPELAND CX Jr, ENNEKING WF: Incidence of osteomyelitis in compound fractures. Am Surg 1965;31:156.

51. EPPS CH Jr, ADAMS JP: Wound management in open fractures. Am Surg 1961;27:766.

52. PATZAKIS MJ, HARVEY JP Jr, IVLER D: The role of antibiotics in the management of open fractures. J Bone Joint Surg 1974;56-A:532.

Chapter 7

UROLOGIC SURGERY

Prophylaxis for urologic operations is a much more complicated matter than in other specialties. The primary issues are twofold:

1. The period of exposure to infection extends beyond the duration of the operation itself, typically because of the risk of the usual indwelling urinary catheter after such operation.
2. The outcome variable is multiple: operative wound infection or postoperative urinary tract infection (or both), with or without fever; and bacteremia.

These and other issues complicate both the conduct and analysis of clinical trials of prophylaxis in urologic surgery. Because bacteria can gain access to the operative site via the indwelling urinary catheter, it is not surprising that the duration of prophylaxis becomes a much more complex issue than in other surgical specialties.

CLINICAL STUDIES AND MICROBIOLOGIC CONSIDERATIONS

In 1938, Gaudin et al.[1] studied the use of sulfanilamide to prevent infection associated with transurethral prostatectomy. They concluded, "Our experience has not demonstrated a sound basis for administration of sulfanilamide in routine postoperative management in these cases." In the ensuing 35 years, the urologic literature has been replete with conflicting reports on the value of antibiotic prophylaxis during prostatectomy. As pointed out by Berger and Nagar[2] in their excellent review, this confusion has resulted from inconsistencies in experimental methodology. The following review and analysis include recent studies, which contain adequate control groups.

111

In a prospective randomized double-blind study, Bogdan[3] evaluated tetracycline prophylaxis for urologic surgery. Sixty-seven patients were given either oral tetracycline or placebo for 11 days beginning immediately postoperatively. The mortality was 6% in both groups. "Minor and major complications" were more common in the placebo group. However, the effect of prophylaxis on bacteriuria and bacteremia was not evaluable, the groups were small, statistical analysis was not performed, and patients with various operative procedures such as suprapubic, retropubic, transurethral, and perineal prostatectomy were included.

One year later, in 1965, Osius et al.[4] published the results of a similar double-blind study using tetracycline prophylaxis. The trial included 88 patients divided into two groups. The first group consisted of 44 patients undergoing diagnostic procedures such as cystoscopy, cystography, and cystometrography. The second group consisted of 44 patients undergoing surgical procedures such as transurethral resection of the prostate (34 patients), transurethral resection of bladder tumor (9 patients), and cystoscopy with litholapaxy (1 patient).

In both the diagnostic and surgical groups, there were no differences noted between tetracycline prophylaxis and placebo[4] in mortality or in preventing postoperative fever, chills, urinary tract infection, and bacteremia. No adverse effects of either tetracycline or placebo were noted. Thus, a 4-day prophylactic course of tetracycline was no better than placebo, an observation that contradicted that of Bogdan,[3] who had used 11 days of tetracycline prophylaxis in the earlier study.

In a subsequent double-blind study of nitrofurantoin prophylaxis in 200 patients undergoing transurethral resection of the prostate, Gross[5] concluded that postoperative urinary tract infection was not prevented, but that prophylaxis prevented postoperative "septicemia." However, infection was not clearly defined in this study, the results of blood cultures were not reported, and statistical analysis was not performed. These and other methodologic flaws impair meaningful interpretation of the data.

In the same year, Kaplan et al.[6] conducted a double-blind study of sulfisoxazole prophylaxis in 71 patients undergoing transurethral resection of the prostate. In contrast to previous studies, prophylaxis was continued for 6 weeks postoperatively. Routine preoperative and postoperative urine cultures and immediately postoperative blood cultures were obtained. Prophylaxis had no effect on the incidence of urinary tract infection at 6 weeks postoperatively (35%

in the sulfisoxazole group vs 22% in the placebo group), postoperative bacteremia (8.6% vs 6%), postoperative fever (34% vs 44%), complications (14% vs 14%), or mortality (3% vs 3%). They concluded that 6 weeks of sulfisoxazole prophylaxis postoperatively had no favorable effect on the outcome of transurethral prostatectomy.

Unlike those earlier investigators, Morris et al.[7] studied only patients with sterile preoperative urine who were undergoing transurethral prostatectomy. One hundred one patients received either placebo or preoperative kanamycin and postoperative co-trimoxazole for 3 weeks. The investigation was prospective but not randomized or blind. Routine preoperative and postoperative (at catheter removal, at discharge, and at follow-up) urine cultures, intraoperative and immediately postoperative (2 hours) blood cultures, and intraoperative prostatic tissue cultures were obtained from patients in both groups. It is of interest that despite negative preoperative urine cultures, most of the prostate tissue cultures were positive for potential pathogens (Table 7–1). Blood cultures were positive in 10 patients, 4 in the antibiotic group (10%) and 6 in the control group (11%). In 6 of the 10 patients (60%), the same organism was recovered from the prostatic tissue cultures. Thus, the incidence of immediately postoperative bacteremia in this series of patients with sterile preoperative urine was 10%; there was a signifi-

Table 7–1. Organisms Cultured from Resected Prostate (Both Groups)

Organism	No. of Cultures	Percentage of Total
Coagulase-positive Staphylococcus	16	22
Coagulase-negative Staphylococcus	14	19
Streptococcus faecalis	11	15
Escherichia coli	8	11
Streptococcus viridans	8	11
Proteus sp.	6	8
Pseudomonas sp.	4	6
Nonhemolytic Streptococcus	3	4
β-hemolytic Streptococcus	1	1
Bacillus sp.	2	3

From Morris et al.,[7] with permission.

cant correlation between the organisms in prostatic tissue and those isolated from operative blood cultures. The three most common pathogens isolated from postoperative urine cultures were *Escherichia coli* (35%), *Streptococcus faecalis* (19%), and *Proteus* sp. (19%) (Table 7–2).

The incidence of positive postoperative urine cultures was significantly reduced from 27% (14/52) to 5% (2/42) by antibiotic prophylaxis. However, the incidence of bacteremia and fever was not significantly different between the two groups. Morris et al.[7] appropriately concluded that in patients with sterile urine preoperatively, antibiotic prophylaxis reduced the incidence of postoperative urinary tract infection but not fever or bacteremia. The authors further advised that patients with infected preoperative urine be treated with an appropriate antibiotic before surgery since there is a fivefold increase in bacteremia in this group. These data are in accord with those presented by Creevy and Feeney[8] in 1954.

Gibbons et al.[9] studied preoperative and postoperative antibiotic prophylaxis in a prospective and randomized but not double-blind trial. Kanamycin was administered until the catheter was removed. Only patients with sterile urine cultures preoperatively were admitted to the trial. Routine blood cultures were not performed. Postoperative bacteremia was reduced from 12% in the control group to 6% in the kanamycin group. However, all 5 "increased-risk" patients were randomized to the control group and became infected. These were patients with neurogenic bladder (1 patient), leukemia (1), or diabetes (1), or those who were receiving steroids (2). Postoperative fever was not affected by prophylaxis, and none of the patients in the study died. The three most common organisms isolated from postoperative urine cultures were *E. coli,* "*Enterococcus,*" and unspeciated *Klebsiella.* The authors concluded that kanamycin prophylaxis was of no value in the uninfected, "non-risk" patients undergoing elective transurethral resection of the prostate. They postulated, however, that high-risk patients (100% infection rate in this series) might benefit from prophylaxis.

Matthew et al.[10] studied nitrofurantoin prophylaxis in 82 patients with sterile urine undergoing transurethral resection of the prostate. The study was prospective and randomized but not double-blind. Forty-seven patients received nitrofurantoin macrocrystals before operation and for 10 days after operation; 40 control patients received no prophylaxis. There were no significant differences in the length of hospitalization (6.4 days in the control group and 7.3 days in the prophylaxis group) or postoperative fever (30% vs

Table 7-2. Significant Organisms Cultured from the Urine (Both Groups)

Organism	Frequency of Culture		Sensitivity to Prophylactic Antibiotics	
	No.	%	No.	%
E. coli	9	35	8	89
S. faecalis	5	19	1	20
Proteus sp.	5	19	4	85
Pseudomonas sp.	1	4	0	0
Coagulase-positive Staphylococcus	3	12	3	100
Coagulase-negative Staphylococcus	1	4	1	100
β-hemolytic Streptococcus	1	4	1	100
Enterobacter sp.	1	4	1	100

Total includes several combined infections.

Modified from Morris et al.,[7] with permission.

21.3%, respectively). The incidence of bacteriuria at 24 hours after catheter removal was reduced from 25% in the control group to 0 in the prophylaxis group; at 1 month postoperatively the rates were 11% and 0, respectively. These differences were statistically significant. Blood cultures were not routinely obtained and bacteremia was therefore not evaluated. None of the patients died.

The three most common bacteria causing postoperative urinary tract infection were *E. coli*, "enterococcus," and unspeciated *Enterobacter*. Matthew et al.[10] concluded that nitrofurantoin prophylaxis for 10 days markedly reduced the incidence of postoperative urinary tract infection. However, they added, "whether to attempt to prevent postoperative bacteriuria in all patients with prophylactic antimicrobials or to treat it when it occurs remains a matter of the surgeon's personal preference."

One well-designed study is that of Nielson et al.,[11] who investigated the use of cefoxitin prophylaxis in 110 patients with sterile urine undergoing transurethral prostatectomy. Urine cultures were obtained at 3 and 7 days postoperatively, and at 4 to 6 weeks postoperatively. Blood cultures were obtained from 10 patients in each group in the recovery room. None of the blood cultures was positive. The incidence of bacteriuria was markedly reduced in the prophylaxis group at 3 days and 7 days. After 7 days, all patients with infected urine were treated with an appropriate antibiotic; thus, at 28 days there were no significant differences between the two groups (Table 7–3). Complications such as fever and epididymitis occurred with equal frequency in the two groups. The authors concluded that cefoxitin prophylaxis after transurethral resection of the prostate markedly reduced the incidence of postoperative bacteriuria, but not fever and other postoperative complications. The most common organism isolated from infected urine was *E. coli*, in accord with the findings of previous authors.

PHARMACOLOGIC CONSIDERATIONS

The choice of drugs for antibacterial prophylaxis in patients undergoing urologic surgery is based on the following premises: (1) high urinary concentrations of the drug, (2) low toxicity, and (3) selective activity of the drug against strains commonly encountered in urinary tract infections.

Table 7-3. Incidence of Infection after Transurethral Resection of the Prostate

	3 Days			7 Days*			28 Days		
	Infected	Uninfected	Totals	Infected	Uninfected	Totals	Infected	Uninfected	Totals
Cefoxitin	2	49	51	3	46	49	3	44	47
Placebo	14	39	53	21	29	50	9	38	47
Significance		$p < 0.005$			$p < 0.0005$			$p < 0.10$	

*After 7 days, all patients with infection (3 in the cefoxitin group and 21 in the placebo group) were treated with an antibiotic other than cefoxitin.

Modified from Nielsen et al,[11] with permission.

Chemoprophylaxis carries the risk of selection of drug-resistant strains that can lead to serious therapeutic problems. The broader the activity spectrum of the drug, the greater the hazard of spread of infections due to drug-resistant strains for which drugs are not readily available.[12]

Successful genitourinary prophylaxis requires adequate tissue concentrations of antibiotic at the target structure. The most frequently used antibiotic groups include sulfonamides, penicillins, tetracyclines, cephalosporins, and aminoglycosides. Renal accumulation of aminoglycosides can lead to toxicity and can be explained in terms of two successive processes: (1) renal tubular reabsorption and (2) electrostatic interaction between the antibiotics and the tissue components. The electrostatic interaction may play an important role in the pathogenesis of aminoglycoside toxicity.[13]

Infection is also an important determinant of renal antibiotic tissue concentration. The intracortical, medullary, and papillary distribution of ampicillin was studied[14] in normal and pyelonephritic rats. At 4 days after induction of pyelonephritis, the animals were given a single injection of 100 mg of ampicillin per kilogram or were treated for 1 week with two doses per day of 100 mg/kg. Major differences in the intrarenal distribution of ampicillin were noted between normal and pyelonephritic animals. At 2 hours after injection, the concentrations of ampicillin in all parts of the infected kidneys were significantly lower ($p < 0.05$) than in normal kidneys. The area under the curve (micrograms times minutes per milliliter) over a 4-hour period after a single injection was much lower in the medulla (6.3 ± 0.9) and papilla (29.6 ± 4.2) of infected kidneys than in the medulla (11.1 ± 1.6) and papilla (43.8 ± 10.1) of noninfected kidneys. Whereas the ratio of concentration in tissue to concentration in serum ranged to 11.1 in the papilla of the normal animals, this ratio was reduced to 2.3 in the pyelonephritic animals. The diminution of the concentration gradient was also striking in the urine: The ratios were reduced by more than three times in pyelonephritic animals. One week of therapy resulted in a noticeable reduction of the inflammatory process, associated with a return to near-normal intrarenal distribution of ampicillin. In normal rats treated with multiple doses, there was a decrease in antibiotic concentration in serum and kidneys and in the area under the time-concentration curve for these tissues.

Moreover, the penetration of antibiotics into prostate tissue varies,[15] and the relation between bacteria in prostatic tissue and coexistent or post-prostatectomy bacteriuria remains unclear.

The appropriate duration for antibiotic prophylaxis is unknown. Administration of antibiotic for 24 hours for specific operations is as effective as a longer course while reducing the frequency of nosocomial infections.[16,17] Unfortunately, the general dictum that short-course prophylaxis, if used at all, is as effective as long-term prophylaxis may not apply to most urologic procedures, which usually are followed by the insertion of catheters that remain in place for many hours or days. However, data to support long-term prophylaxis for these surgical procedures are lacking. Furthermore, overzealous prolongation of prophylaxis may significantly increase the incidence of nosocomial urinary tract infections.[18–21]

Lacy et al.,[22] using long-term cephaloridine prophylaxis, found an infection rate of 28% after prostatectomy. In their control group, the infection rate was 62.5%. In contrast, Shah et al.[23] used short-term cephalexin prophylaxis and found their infection rate to be 16%. This three-dose regimen, therefore, was more effective than that of Lacy et al., who used prophylaxis for a mean of 7.6 days. Thus, short-term antibiotic regimens decreased urinary tract infection rates after prostatectomy and reduced the possibility of emergence of antibiotic-resistant organisms. Short regimens are inexpensive and are associated with few side effects; in addition, patients are not required to continue antibiotic treatment after discharge.

The use of postoperative irrigation with antiseptic solutions has also been investigated and has yielded conflicting results. Bastable et al.[24] reported a postoperative urinary tract infection rate of 50% with saline irrigation. However, in a study by Shah et al.[23] there was an infection rate of 28% in the control group with routine saline irrigation postoperatively.

PRACTICAL SURGICAL RECOMMENDATIONS

Review of the literature supports the following conclusions and recommendations:

1. Patients with infected urine who are undergoing transurethral prostatectomy should be treated with an appropriate antibiotic before surgery; there is a fivefold increase in bacteremia in untreated patients with infected urine who undergo prostatic surgery.

2. In patients with sterile urine, antibiotic prophylaxis reduces the incidence of postoperative urinary tract infection; however, bacteremia, fever, and other urologic complications are unaffected by prophylaxis in this group of patients.
3. Overall mortality is unaffected by antibiotic prophylaxis for prostatic surgery.
4. An antibiotic selected for patients undergoing urologic surgery should produce high urinary and urinary tract tissue concentrations, should have low toxicity, and should be effective against strains commonly encountered in urinary tract infections.
5. The duration of prophylaxis and its costs and benefits in patients with sterile urine preoperatively have not been clearly defined and therefore require further careful clinical investigation. Short-term antibiotic regimens seem to produce fewer antibiotic-resistant organisms, are inexpensive, and are associated with fewer untoward effects.
6. The use of postoperative irrigation with antiseptic solutions is probably no more effective than routine irrigation with saline solution.

REFERENCES

1. GAUDIN HJ, ZIDE HA, THOMPSON GJ: Use of sulfanilamide after transurethral prostatectomy. JAMA 1938;110:1887.
2. BERGER SA, NAGAR H: Antimicrobial prophylaxis in urology. J Urol 1978;120:319.
3. BOGDAN PE: The value of prophylactic tetracycline therapy after prostatic surgery: Interim report of a double-blind study. J Am Geriatr Soc 1964;12:977.
4. OSIUS TG, TAVEL FR, HINMAN F Jr: Tetracycline used prophylactically in transurethral procedures. Maryland Med J 1965;14:37.
5. GROSS M: Use of an antimicrobial agent to prevent complications following transurethral resection of the prostate: Furandantin. Int Surg 1969;51:475.
6. KAPLAN GW, BELMAN AB, KROPP KA: A double blind study of sulfa prophylaxis after transurethral resection. Invest Urol 1969;7:181.

7. MORRIS MJ, GOLOVSKY D, GUINNESS MDG et al: The value of prophylactic antibiotics in transurethral prostatic resection: A controlled trial, with observations on the origin of postoperative infection. Br J Urol 1976;48:479.

8. CREEVY CD, FEENEY MJ: Routine use of antibiotics in transurethral prostatic resection: Clinical investigation. J Urol 1954; 71:615.

9. GIBBONS RP, STARK RA, CORREA RJ Jr et al: The prophylactic use—or misuse—of antibiotics in transurethral prostatectomy. J Urol 1978;119:381.

10. MATTHEW AD, GONZALEZ R, JEFFORDS D et al: Prevention of bacteriuria after transurethral prostatectomy with nitrofurantoin macrocrystals. J Urol 1978;120:442.

11. NIELSEN OS, MAIGAARD S, FRIMODT-MØLLER N et al: Prophylactic antibiotics in transurethral prostatectomy. J Urol 1981; 126:60.

12. WESOLOWSKI S, WENCEL J, CZAPLICKI M et al: Antibacterial prophylaxis in patients after prostatectomy. Int Urol Nephrol 1977;9:241.

13. KOMIYA I, UMEMURA K, FUJITA M et al: Mechanism of renal distribution of aminoglycoside antibiotics. J Pharm Dyn 1980;3:299.

14. TROTTIER S, BERGERON MG: Intrarenal concentrations of ampicillin in acute pyelonephritis. Antimicrob Agents Chemother 1981;19:761.

15. STAMEY TA, MEARES EM Jr, WINNINGHAM DG: Chronic bacterial prostatitis and the diffusion of drugs into prostatic fluid. J Urol 1970;103:187.

16. DOWNING R, McLEISH AR, BURDON DW et al: Duration of systemic prophylactic antibiotic cover against anaerobic sepsis in intestinal surgery. Dis Colon Rectum 1977;20:401.

17. STONE HH, HOOPER CA, KOLB LD et al: Antibiotic prophylaxis in gastric, biliary and colonic surgery. Ann Surg 1976; 184:443.

18. GARIBALDI RA, BURKE JP, DICKMAN ML et al: Factors predisposing to bacteriuria during indwelling urethral catheterization. N Engl J Med 1974;291:215.

19. KERESTECI AG, LEERS WD: Indwelling catheter infection. Can Med Assoc J 1973;109:711.

20. ORR LM, DANIEL WR, CAMPBELL JL et al: Effect of nitrofurantoin (furadantin) on morbidity after transurethral prostatic resection. JAMA 1958;167:1455.

21. PETERSDORF RG, CURTIN JA, HOEPRICH PD et al: A study of antibiotic prophylaxis in unconscious patients. N Engl J Med 1975;257:1001.
22. LACY SS, DRACH GW, COX CE: Incidence of infection after prostatectomy and efficacy of cephaloridine prophylaxis. J Urol 1971;105:836.
23. SHAH PJR, WILLIAMS G, CHAUDARY M: Short-term antibiotic prophylaxis and prostatectomy. Br J Urol 1981;53:339.
24. BASTABLE JR, PEEL RN, BIRCH DM et al: Continuous irrigation of the bladder after prostatectomy: Its effect on post-prostatectomy infection. Br J Urol 1977;49:689.

Chapter 8

NEUROSURGERY

Defining the role (or nonrole, as the case may be) of antibiotic prophylaxis in neurosurgical practice has been difficult. Many craniotomies are inherently not only clean procedures but are classically "refined" or very clean; this eventuates in a low infection rate, in part because of the rich blood supply to the head and neck area, but also because of the absence of endogenous microbial contamination in those instances. Carefully conducted trials of infection in neurosurgery are few.[1]

In 1974, Savitz et al.[2] reported the results of an uncontrolled trial of antibiotic prophylaxis in neurosurgical patients. When ampicillin was administered prophylactically during a 12-month period, the wound infection rate was 5.1%. During the subsequent 12 months, lincomycin given prophylactically reduced the wound infection rate to 2.3%. This difference was not statistically significant ($p > 0.1$).

On the basis of these data, Savitz and Malis[3] conducted a randomized double-blind trial comparing perioperative use of clindamycin with placebo. Although the authors intended to carry out the study for 1 year, it was interrupted in the sixth month when an epidemic of postoperative wound infections occurred during a period of increased surgical scheduling. Of seven craniotomies that became infected during the epidemic period, six were in patients who received placebo, and one was in a patient who received clindamycin. During the earlier nonepidemic period, three wound infections occurred in 33 patients who received placebo, but none occurred in 56 patients who received clindamycin.

Causes of infections and deaths in both of these studies[2,3] are summarized in Table 8–1. Infection was due predominantly to staphylococci and aerobic gram-negative rods. All 3 deaths, 2 in the 1974 study and 1 in the 1976 study, were related to gram-negative wound infections (one *Escherichia coli,* one unspeciated *Klebsiella,* and one unspeciated *Pseudomonas*).

Table 8–1. Causes of Infection

Patient Regimen	Gram-Positive Organisms (No. of Infections)	Gram-Negative Organisms (No. of Infections)
Placebo	*Staphylococcus* (6): *aureus* (4) *albus* (2)	*E. coli* (1) (death)
Antibiotics	*Staphylococcus* (5): *aureus* (3) *albus* (1) *epidermidis* (1)	*Proteus* (3): *mirabilis* (2) *morganii* (1) *Klebsiella* (1) (death) *Pseudomonas* (1) (death) *E. coli* (1) *Bacteroides* (1) *Serratia* (1)

Modified from Savitz and Malis,[3] with permission.

The authors[2,3] concluded that perioperative clindamycin was effective in reducing wound infection rates in neurosurgical patients who had undergone prolonged operations (longer than 6 hours) or reexploration. As pointed out by Haines,[4] however, the epidemic of infections occurring during a 2-week period of increased surgical load skews the data and prevents valid statistical analysis.

In a subsequent (1979) retrospective analysis of 1,732 major clean neurosurgical procedures,[5] there were no postoperative wound infections. All patients received tobramycin or gentamicin intramuscularly, vancomycin intravenously, and a streptomycin irrigating solution. The total absence of wound infection in such a large number of major procedures is unprecedented. However, important details are omitted from the report and follow-up data are not included. Therefore, the efficacy of this regimen requires confirmation in a controlled trial.

Savitz and Katz[6] reported similar results after instituting routine antistaphylococcal prophylaxis in three community hospitals. All patients received either methicillin when foreign materials, such as shunts, were inserted or cephalothin. Patients who were allergic to penicillin received erythromycin. No cases of primary wound infections were encountered in 1,000 consecutive cases. Two patients, both of whom survived, suffered delayed extracranial infections (one due to unspeciated *Klebsiella* and one due to unspeciated *Pseudomonas*), further complicated by meningitis.

Thus, in the setting of a community hospital, antistaphylococcal prophylaxis for neurosurgical procedures resulted in a remarkably low postoperative infection rate—similar to that reported earlier by Malis.[5] These important results, however, require confirmation by controlled investigation.

Ajir et al.[7] reviewed their experience with prophylactic methicillin to prevent infection in cerebrospinal fluid shunts. This study was retrospective and used historical controls. There were 8 infections in 105 procedures done without prophylaxis (7.6%) and 3 infections in 66 procedures done with prophylaxis (4.5%). This difference was not statistically significant (Table 8–2).

Of 32 patients who had shunt revisions without prophylactic methicillin, 4 became infected (12.5%); of 32 done with prophylaxis, none became infected. This difference was statistically significant. Thus, prophylaxis in this study[7] appeared effective in reducing the rate of shunt infection after revision but not after primary implantation.

Of a total of 11 shunt infections, 2 were due to coagulase-negative staphylococci, 3 to coagulase-positive staphylococci, 3 to *Pseudomonas aeruginosa,* 2 to *Klebsiella pneumoniae,* and 1 to *Proteus* sp. plus *E. coli.*

Methodologic flaws in that study[7] prevent the drawing of firm conclusions regarding the efficacy of prophylaxis for shunt procedures. Similarly, other previously published reports[8–13] are retrospective, not randomized, have too few patients, have poor microbiologic or clinical follow-up, or have other serious design flaws.

There are no adequately designed trials that examine the use of

Table 8–2. Infection Rates for Procedures with or without Prophylactic Methicillin

	No. of Procedures	No. of Infections	Percentage of Infection
Without methicillin	105	8	7.61
Primary VP shunt placement	73	4	5.48
VP shunt revision	32	4	12.5
With methicillin	66	3	4.54
Primary VP shunt placement	34	3	8.82
VP shunt revision	32	0	0

VP, ventriculoperitoneal.

Modified from Ajir et al.,[7] with permission.

antibiotic prophylaxis for cranioplasty, external ventriculostomy, or transsphenoidal hypophysectomy.

The use of antibiotic prophylaxis for patients with skull fracture with or without leakage of cerebrospinal fluid is controversial. Studies[14-20] are retrospective or involve consecutively treated patients without adequate controls.

In a randomized trial, Hoff et al.[21] investigated the use of penicillin prophylaxis for patients with basilar skull fracture without cerebrospinal fluid leakage. No infections occurred in 160 patients, and the authors concluded that prophylaxis in such patients was not useful. Klastersky et al.[22] came to a similar conclusion in a placebo-controlled double-blind evaluation of penicillin prophylaxis in 52 patients with cerebrospinal leakage. These last two studies may have examined too few patients to detect differences between prophylaxis and placebo.[23]

The issue of wound infection must be separated from infection involving implanted devices. Neurosurgical prostheses—particularly shunts for hydrocephalus—are frequently contaminated as a consequence of surgically unrelated or spontaneous bacteremia; such delayed contamination and infection would be unlikely to respond well to perioperative prophylaxis. The role of chronic prophylactic regimens in such patients has not been studied. A final conclusion as to the merits of perioperative antibiotic use is more difficult today in neurosurgery than in its related disciplines. Conceptually, prophylaxis with *safe* agents, including antistaphylococcal activity, is probably justified when infection rates can be expected to exceed 2%.

CONCLUSIONS AND PRACTICAL SURGICAL RECOMMENDATIONS

1. There are no persuasive data as to the value of routine antibiotic use in basilar skull fractures.
2. In elective craniotomy, no evidence exists to support the routine use of systemic antibiotic prophylaxis. However, if such an agent is used, its spectrum should be primarily antistaphylococcal.
3. In elective craniotomy involving implantable prosthetic devices, for example, cranioplasty and shunt placement, perioperative prophylaxis with an agent such as nafcillin, 1

g intravenously, before and after operation is justified in adults. This is especially sound when reoperation is required.

4. No data are available pertinent to chronic antibiotic prophylaxis in patients with shunts in place for hydrocephalus. Dental and other procedures likely to produce bacteremia in such patients may justify systemic antibiotic prophylaxis administered before the procedure.

5. The use of antibiotic prophylaxis in transsphenoidal hypophysectomy has not been studied.

REFERENCES

1. WRIGHT RL, BURKE JF: Effect of ultraviolet radiation on postoperative sepsis. J Neurosurg 1969;31:533.
2. SAVITZ MH, MALIS LI, MEYERS BR: Prophylactic antibiotics in neurosurgery. Surg Neurol 1974;2:95.
3. SAVITZ MH, MALIS LI: Prophylactic clindamycin for neurosurgical patients. NY State J Med 1976;76:64.
4. HAINES SJ: Systemic antibiotic prophylaxis in neurological surgery. Neurosurgery 1980;6:355.
5. MALIS LI: Prevention of neurosurgical infection by intraoperative antibiotics. Neurosurgery 1979;5:339.
6. SAVITZ MH, KATZ SS: Rationale for prophylactic antibiotics in neurosurgery. Neurosurgery 1981;9:142.
7. AJIR F, LEVIN AB, DUFF TA: Effect of prophylactic methicillin on cerebrospinal fluid shunt infections in children. Neurosurgery 1981;9:6.
8. TSINGOGLOU S, FORREST DM: A technique for the insertion of Holter ventriculo-atrial shunt for infantile hydrocephalus. Br J Surg 1971;58:367.
9. YU HC, PATTERSON RH Jr: Prophylactic antimicrobial agents after ventriculoatriostomy for hydrocephalus. J Pediatr Surg 1973;8:881.
10. McLAURIN RL: Infected cerebrospinal fluid shunts. Surg Neurol 1973;1:191.
11. SCHOENBAUM SC, GARDNER P, SHILLITO J: Infections of cerebrospinal fluid shunts: Epidemiology, clinical manifestations, and therapy. J Infect Dis 1975;131:543.
12. NAITO H, TOYA S, SHIZAWA H et al: High incidence of acute postoperative meningitis and septicemia in patients undergo-

ing craniotomy with ventriculoatrial shunt. Surg Gynecol Obstet 1973;137:810.

13. WEISS SR, RASKIND R: Further experience with the ventriculoperitoneal shunt: Prophylactic antibiotics. Int Surg 1970;53:300.

14. LEECH P: Cerebrospinal fluid leakage, dural fistulae and meningitis after basal skull fractures. Injury 1974;6:141.

15. BRAWLEY BW, KELLEY WA: Treatment of basal skull fractures with and without cerebrospinal fluid fistulae. J Neurosurg 1967;26:57.

16. RAAF J; Posttraumatic cerebrospinal fluid leaks. Arch Surg 1967;95:648.

17. OMMAYA AK: Spinal fluid fistulae. Clin Neurosurg 1975; 23:363.

18. MacGEE EE, CAUTHEN JC, BRACKETT CE: Meningitis following acute traumatic cerebrospinal fluid fistula. J Neurosurg 1970; 33:312.

19. RASKIND R, DORIA A: Cerebrospinal fluid rhinorrhea and otorrhea of traumatic origin. Int Surg 1966;46:223.

20. IGNELZI RJ, VanderARK GD: Analysis of the treatment of basilar skull fractures with and without antibiotics. J Neurosurg 1975;43:721.

21. HOFF JT, BREWIN A, U HS: Antibiotics for basilar skull fracture. J Neurosurg 1976;44:649 (Letter).

22. KLASTERSKY J, SADEGHI M, BRIHAYE J: Antimicrobial prophylaxis in patients with rhinorrhea or otorrhea: A double-blind study. Surg Neurol 1976;6:111.

23. FREIMAN JA, CHALMERS TC, SMITH H Jr et al: The importance of beta, the type II error and sample size in the design and interpretation of the randomized control trial: Survey of 71 "negative" trials. N Engl J Med 1978;299:690.

Chapter 9
HEAD AND NECK
SURGERY

Otolaryngologic and other major head and neck procedures present problems of analysis similar to those associated with other operations performed by general surgeons. Some clean operations in a richly vascularized area are unlikely to benefit from systemic prophylactic antibiotics. As is the case with procedures involving entrance into a contaminated viscus, prophylaxis is effective when radical surgery is combined with entry into the oral cavity, pharynx, or larynx.

The controversy over the value of antibiotic prophylaxis for head and neck and otolaryngologic surgery is as persistent and unsettled as it is in other subspecialties.

In 1961, King[1] denounced the use of prophylaxis in head and neck surgery:

> It seems that under ordinary circumstances, the following conclusions are justifiable: 1. The usefulness of antibiotic prophylaxis has not been proven. 2. The expense is great, and when multiplied by many hospital admissions, becomes astronomical. 3. The public health problem is increasing and will continue to do so. 4. Toxic and allergic reactions are common. 5. The basic usefulness of antibiotics is being destroyed by indiscriminate prophylactic use.

Two years later, Strong[2] reviewed the incidence of postoperative infection in 287 patients undergoing otolaryngologic procedures without antibiotic prophylaxis. The infection rate was 2.4%. The author concluded that this rate approached that found in other "clean" surgical procedures and was not likely to be reduced further by antibiotic prophylaxis.

In contrast to these conclusions, Ketcham et al.[3,4] published reports in 1962 and 1963, which indicated that prophylaxis was effective in head and neck surgery. However, each of these studies included cancer surgery at various anatomic sites. The fraction of patients undergoing head and neck procedures was small and was not subjected to statistical analysis.

In a similar investigation using prophylactic cephaloridine, Brown et al.[5] studied 182 patients undergoing general surgical procedures. In 21 of 92 patients in the placebo group and in 6 of 90 in the cephaloridine group, infectious complications developed, that is, wound infection, pulmonary infection or urinary tract infection. This difference was statistically significant ($p < 0.01$). However, only 18 of the 182 patients described underwent head and neck surgery. In this small subgroup, there was no significant difference in results between cephaloridine prophylaxis and placebo. Similar results were obtained by Evans and Pollock,[6] who used cephaloridine in 762 patients undergoing different general surgical procedures. Again, in a small subgroup of 20 patients undergoing head and neck procedures, there was no significant difference in results between cephaloridine prophylaxis and placebo.

Two double-blind studies, one by Dor and Klastersky[7] and the other by Becker and Parell,[8] evaluated the efficacy of antibiotic prophylaxis in patients undergoing surgery for head and neck cancer. Both groups of investigators concluded that prophylaxis was beneficial in this group of patients.

Dor and Klastersky[7] studied 102 patients, 52 of whom received ampicillin and cloxacillin, 2 g of each daily, beginning 1 day preoperatively and continuing for 5 days postoperatively, and 50 of whom received placebo. Patients were stratified according to the extent of surgery; procedures were classified as either minor, moderately extensive, or very extensive.

The incidence of postoperative infection,[7] by group, is summarized in Table 9–1. Eighteen of 50 patients in the placebo group and 9 of 52 in the prophylaxis group became infected. This difference was statistically significant ($p < 0.05$). In both the placebo and prophylaxis groups, the incidence of infection increased with the severity of the surgery. Thus, with minor procedures the infection rate was 11.1% in the placebo group and 7.7% in the prophylaxis group. With very extensive surgery, over half the patients (54.5%) in the placebo group and more than one third of patients (36.4%) in the prophylaxis group became infected.

Gram-negative rods, particularly *Pseudomonas aeruginosa, Proteus mirabilis,* and the *Klebsiella–Enterobacter–Serratia* group, were isolated from 14 of the 18 infected patients in the placebo group, and from 8 of 9 infected patients in the prophylaxis group.[7] *Staphylococ-*

Table 9–1. Incidence of Postoperative Wound Infection in Patients Receiving Antibiotic Prophylaxis or Placebo

	Placebo			Ampicillin + Cloxacillin		
		Infections			Infections	
Type of Surgical Operation	No. of Cases	No.	%	No. of Cases	No.	%
Minor	9	1	11.1	13	1	7.7
Moderately extensive	30	11	36.6	28	4	14.3
Very extensive	11	6	54.4	11	4	36.4
Total*	50	18	36.0	52	9	17.3

*$p < 0.05$; $\chi^2 = 4.81$.

From Dor and Klastersky,[7] with permission.

cus aureus, alone or in mixed infection, was isolated from 7 of the 18 infected patients in the placebo group and from 3 of 9 infected patients in the prophylaxis group. The distribution of these organisms between the placebo and prophylaxis groups is similar. Thus, prophylaxis in this series[7] appeared to have little effect on the bacteriology of the primary infection. In addition, the antibiotic sensitivities of all bacterial strains were determined; increased resistance was not demonstrable in the organisms isolated from infected patients in the prophylaxis group.

Anaerobes are commonly found in infection after head and neck surgery.[9] Since none was described by Dor and Klastersky,[7] anaerobic isolation techniques probably were not used.

Becker and Parell[8] studied prophylactic cefazolin in 55 patients undergoing head and neck surgery for cancer. They included only patients in whom the upper aerodigestive tract was entered from the neck. These were patients in whom the operative field would be contaminated by a rich aerobic and anaerobic normal flora and in whom the expected infection rate would be high.[9] The study[8] was prospective, randomized, and double-blind. Cultures of multiple sites were obtained routinely before, during, and after operation. Wound infections were cultured aerobically and anaerobically. Cefazolin or placebo was given 2 hours (intramuscularly) or 1 hour (intravenously) preoperatively and was continued postoperatively every 6 hours for 24 hours (Table 9–2).

Twelve of 32 patients (38%) who received cefazolin and 20 of 23 (87%) who received placebo became infected.[8] This difference was highly significant ($p < 0.001$). The extraordinarily high risk of postoperative infection in this group of patients and the value of prophylaxis are confirmed by these observations. Further analysis of the data indicated that the patients who benefited most from prophylaxis were those who had intraoral procedures with radical or modified neck dissection.

The authors[8] found that preoperative and intraoperative cultures helped in determining which anaerobic organisms would be isolated postoperatively. *Bacteroides fragilis,* however, was not

Table 9–2. Infection Rates in Cefazolin and Placebo Groups

	Cefazolin	Placebo
Number of patients	32	23
Number of patients infected	12 (38%)	20 (87%)
	$p < 0.001$	

From Becker and Parell,[8] with permission.

isolated from any cultures. The single most common pathogen was *S. aureus*, which was isolated from 9 of 30 (30%) infections. Gram-negative rods were isolated from 11 of 30 (37%) infected patients. The preponderant aerobic gram-negative organisms were *Haemophilus influenzae* and *Klebsiella pneumoniae*.

In a later study, Becker et al.[9] defined the full range of aerobic and anaerobic flora isolated from wound infection after head and neck surgery (Tables 9–3 and 9–4).

Eschelman et al.[10] conducted a prospective, double-blind study

Table 9–3. Aerobic Bacteria Cultured from Infected Wounds

Gram-Positive	Gram-Negative
β-*Streptococcus* (group A)	*Eikenella corrodens*
β-*Streptococcus* (not group A)	*Haemophilus influenzae*
α-*Streptococcus*	*Haemophilus parainfluenzae*
γ-*Streptococcus*	*Moraxella* sp.
Group D *Streptococcus*	*Neisseria* sp.
Microaerophilic *Streptococcus*	*Enterobacter aerogenes*
Staphylococcus aureus	*Enterobacter cloacae*
Staphylococcus epidermidis	*Klebsiella pneumoniae*
Corynebacterium sp.	*Proteus mirabilis*
	Pseudomonas aeruginosa

Modified from Becker et al.,[9] with permission.

Table 9–4. Anaerobic Bacteria Cultured from Infected Wounds

Gram-positive cocci	Gram-negative rods
Peptococcus asaccharolyticus	*Bacteroides amylophilus*
P. magnus	*B. capillosus*
P. prevotii	*B. disiens*
P. variabilis	*B. melaninogenicus* sp.
Peptostreptococcus anaerobius	*B. melaninogenicus*
P. micros	(subsp. *intermedius*)
Gram-positive rods	*B. melaninogenicus*
Actinomyces sp.	(subsp. *melaninogenicus*)
A. viscosus	*B. oralis*
Bifidobacterium sp.	*B. ruminicola* (subsp. *brevis*)
Eubacterium sp.	*Bacteroides* sp.
Lactobacillus catenaforme	*Fusobacterium aquatile*
L. delbrueckii	*F. necrophorum*
L. minutus	*F. nucleatum*
Lactobacillus sp.	Gram-negative cocci
Propionibacterium acnes	*Veillonella alcalescens*
Propionibacterium sp.	*Acidaminococcus fermentans*
	V. parvula

From Becker et al.,[9] with permission.

of antibiotic prophylaxis in otolaryngologic procedures. They compared penicillin, ampicillin, and placebo in 330 patients undergoing tympanoplasty, mastoidectomy, rhinoplasty, Caldwell-Luc operation, and plastic surgery. The series included 28 patients who underwent major head and neck surgery with or without entry into the oral cavity or pharynx. The authors concluded that prophylaxis was of no value in general otolaryngologic surgery except in those head and neck procedures that involved entry into the aerodigestive tract. Their conclusions confirmed those of Becker and Parell.[8]

PHARMACOLOGIC CONSIDERATIONS

If we assume that prophylaxis is warranted in patients undergoing extensive surgery for head and neck cancer, the selection of antibiotic and the time and duration of prophylaxis are crucial in preventing postoperative infections. Prolonged antibiotic administration, whether for treatment or prophylaxis, is costly, can produce an increased frequency and severity of adverse reactions, and carries a greater risk of superinfections.

Mombelli et al.[11] compared short-term (1 day) with long-term (4 days) carbenicillin prophylaxis in patients undergoing head and neck cancer operations. Prolonged administration did not offer an advantage over the 1-day regimen. There was a trend toward higher frequency and severity of hypokalemia among patients who received the prolonged prophylaxis. Another unfavorable consequence in this latter group was the higher rate of wound colonization by *Klebsiella* sp.

As already mentioned, wound infections after major head and neck cancer surgery are often polymicrobial. Broad-spectrum penicillins such as carbenicillin, ticarcillin, and piperacillin could theoretically be used because of their activity against gram-positive, gram-negative, and most anaerobic microorganisms, all of which can be responsible for wound infections after such operations.

Combination antibiotic prophylaxis has also been investigated. Clark et al.[12] used ampicillin and cloxacillin, given intravenously before the initial incision, repeated every 2 hours during surgery, and administered postoperatively every 4 to 6 hours for 96 hours. Ampicillin was selected for its broad spectrum and cloxacillin for its antistaphylococcal activity.

Becker[13] has recommended cefazolin for prophylaxis because of its effectiveness against aerobic pathogens most commonly isolated from infected wounds and anaerobic bacteria normally residing in the oropharynx. Cefazolin was administered 1 g preoperatively and 0.5 g every 6 hours for 4 doses. With this regimen, appropriate tissue levels were achieved before bacterial intraoperative wound contamination occurred, and they were maintained until bacterial contamination was presumably over.

PRACTICAL RECOMMENDATIONS

There is still debate as to the drug of choice and the duration of prophylaxis. The clearest studies seem to parallel general surgical observations: (1) A short, perioperative course of cephalosporin should be used, for example, cefazolin 0.5 g before operation and then 0.5 g after operation, for a maximum of three doses. (2) Antibiotic prophylaxis is effective only in surgery in which the expected postoperative infection rates are high, that is, procedures that involve entry into the aerodigestive tract. (3) Certain otologic and laryngologic reconstructive procedures, especially involving implants, should probably be similarly managed, though adequate data are not available.

REFERENCES

1. KING GD: The case against antibiotic prophylaxis in major head and neck surgery. Laryngoscope 1961;71:647.
2. STRONG MS: Wound infection in otolaryngologic surgery and the inexpediency of antibiotic prophylaxis. Laryngoscope 1963;73:165.
3. KETCHAM AS, BLOCH JH, CRAWFORD DT et al: The role of prophylactic antibiotic therapy in control of staphylococcal infections following cancer surgery. Surg Gynecol Obstet 1962;114:345.
4. KETCHAM AS, LIEBERMAN JE, WEST JT: Antibiotic prophylaxis in cancer surgery and its value in staphylococcal carrier patients. Surg Gynecol Obstet 1963;117:1.

5. BROWN JW, COOPER N, RAMBO WM: Controlled prospective double-blind evaluation of a "prophylactic" antibiotic (cephaloridine) in surgery. Antimicrob Agents Chemother 1969;421-423.

6. EVANS C, POLLOCK AV: The reduction of surgical wound infections by prophylactic parenteral cephaloridine. Br J Surg 1973;60:434.

7. DOR P, KLASTERSKY J: Prophylactic antibiotics in oral, pharyngeal and laryngeal surgery for cancer: A double-blind study. Laryngoscope 1973;83, 1992.

8. BECKER GD, PARELL GJ: Cefazolin prophylaxis in head and neck cancer surgery. Ann Otol Rhinol Laryngol 1979;88 (Pt 1):183.

9. BECKER GD, PARELL J, BUSCH DF et al: Anaerobic and aerobic bacteriology in head and neck cancer surgery. Arch Otolargyngol 1978;104:591.

10. ESCHELMAN LT, SCHLEUNING AJ II, BRUMMETT RE: Prophylactic antibiotics in otolaryngologic surgery: A double-blind study. Trans Am Acad Ophthalmol Otolaryngol 1971; 75:387.

11. MOMBELLI G, COPPENS L, DOR P et al: Antibiotic prophylaxis in surgery for head and neck cancer: Comparative study of short and prolonged administration of carbenicillin. J Antimicrob Agents Chemother 1981;7:665.

12. CLARK GM, PYMAN BC, PAVILLARD RE: A protocol for the prevention of infection in cochlear implant surgery. J Laryngol Otol 1980;94:1377.

13. BECKER GD: Chemoprophylaxis for surgery of the head and neck. Ann Otol Rhinol Laryngol 1981;90:8.

Chapter **10**

OBSTETRICS AND GYNECOLOGY

Ronald S. Gibbs

Soon after antibiotics became commercially available, studies appeared concerning prophylaxis during childbirth. As we have refined our knowledge of risks and benefits, interest has generally centered on procedures with a high risk of postoperative infection.

The use of antibiotic prophylaxis in an obstetric-gynecologic population may be different from its use in other surgical patients: First, nearly all obstetric and most gynecologic patients are healthy and free of serious, underlying disorders. Second, although the lower genital tract is a field contaminated with various aerobic and anaerobic species, gram-negative organisms resistant to multiple antibiotics are not found except under particular circumstances. Third, operation through or adjacent to this contaminated field leads to a moderate to high incidence of infection, but serious infection, such as bacteremia or abscess, or death is unusual. Finally, certain antimicrobials for prophylaxis in pregnancy are contraindicated because of the possibility of adverse effects on the fetus, the newborn, or the mother.

USES OF PROPHYLAXIS IN OBSTETRICS

Cesarean Delivery

Throughout the United States, there has been an unprecedented rise in the incidence of cesarean births within the last two decades. In California, the percentage of births by cesarean section increased from 5% in 1960 to 13% in 1975.[1] Recent data from the National

137

Center for Health Statistics[2] show that for 1978 cesarean sections comprised 15.2% of all deliveries. This rise has been largely attributed to avoidance of potentially traumatic breech or forceps deliveries.[2] In some hospitals, the use of fetal monitoring has also led to a higher rate of cesarean deliveries performed because of fetal distress. A recent conference sponsored by the National Institutes of Health addressed many problems raised by this increase in the cesarean birth rate.[3]

At the same time, it has been recognized that cesarean delivery is accompanied by more frequent and more serious puerperal infections.[4] Indeed, cesarean delivery is probably the greatest single risk factor for maternal postpartum infection. The risk of infection after cesarean delivery is 5 to 30 times greater than after vaginal delivery.[4]

Not all cesarean sections carry the same risk of puerperal infection. Investigators have found that patients in labor with membrane rupture are at greater risk with cesarean section than patients having electively scheduled procedures.[5] Especially among indigent populations, the risk in this subgroup has been reported to be 45% to 85%. Labor, duration of membrane rupture, and repeated vaginal examinations increase postpartum infection, probably because they allow ascent of bacteria into the amniotic cavity before surgery. One might consider this a subclinical infection established while the patient is in labor.[6,7]

Since 1968, nearly 30 studies have been reported on the use of prophylactic antibiotics in cesarean section. The results in randomized trials[8–23] are shown in Table 10–1. With few exceptions, prophylactic regimens resulted in a statistically significant and clinically meaningful decrease in postoperative infection. Polk[24] reported that in 15 randomized placebo-controlled clinical trials of primary cesarean deliveries, the overall preventive fraction

$$\frac{\text{Infection rate in placebo group} - \text{infection rate in prophylaxis group}}{\text{Infection rate in placebo group}}$$

with prophylaxis was 55% of infections. These significant decreases in infection are attributed mainly to decreases in endomyometritis and in wound infections. Urinary tract infections, including both symptomatic and asymptomatic disorders, occurred less commonly in combined series (13% in control subjects vs. 6% in the prophylactic group)[25] but there were significant decreases in only a few individual studies.

Four studies compared the efficacy of antibiotics: Itskovitz et al.[26] compared ampicillin with cephalothin; Kreutner et al.[16] compared cephalothin with cefamandole; Vaughn[27] compared

Table 10–1. Results of Randomized Placebo-Controlled Trials of Antibiotic Prophylaxis in Patients Undergoing Cesarean Section

Author	Antibiotic Regimen (Doses)	No. of Patients	Postoperative Infection Rate[†] Placebo Group (%)	Prophylyaxis Group (%)
Gibbs[8]	Ampicillin, kanamycin, and methicillin (3)	61	42	21
Gibbs[9]	Ampicillin and kanamycin (3)	68	64*	17*
Work[10]	Cephalothin (3)	80	42.5*	20*
Wong[11]	Cefazolin (3)	93	58*	35*
Kreutner[12]	Cefazolin (3)	97	26	16
Gall[13]	Cefazolin or cephalothin (4)	95	37*	13*
Phelan[14]	Cefazolin (3)	122	16	11
Larson[15]	Cefoxitin (3)	152	33*	19*
Kreutner[16]	Cephalothin or cefamandole (2)	120	59*	30*
Duff[17]	Ampicillin (3)	57	42*	8*
McCowan[18]	Metronidazole (2)	73	31	37
Rehu[19]	Penicillin or clindamycin and gentamicin (1)	147	33*	8*
Harger[20]	Cefoxitin (3)	386	27.5*	11*
Polk[21]	Cefoxitin (3)	266	20*	4*
Dillon[22]	Cefoxitin (3)	101	29*	4*
Gibbs[23]	Cefamandole (3)	100	52*	16*
Stiver[28]	Cefoxitin or cefazolin (3)	354	24.3*	6*

*Significant difference in infection rate, by χ^2 test.

† Infections noted are of the operative site, when information was provided by authors.

cephradine with metronidazole; and Rehu and Jahkola[19] compared penicillin with clindamycin plus gentamicin. None of these trials showed a statistically significant difference in infection rates. However, the populations in these studies were small (88-118), and the absolute differences in infection rate were also small (3%-8%). In addition, Stiver et al.[28] compared cefoxitin with cefazolin in non-elective cesarean section. They found no significant differences with regard to genital tract infections or hospital stay.

Studies comparing short with long courses are few. D'Angelo and Sokol[29] carried out a randomized clinical trial with cephalo-sporin, comparing a 24-hour regimen with a 5-day regimen. They found no significant difference in the rate of postoperative infection (29% for the short course, compared with 20% for the long course). In Nigeria, Ayangade[30] found that a course of 6 to 10 days was accompanied by more postoperative fever (41%) than was a 12-

hour course (10%), but this was not a randomized study. Swartz and Grolle,[25] combining data from 26 studies, concluded that regimens of 12 hours or less are as effective as longer prophylactic courses.

Studies comparing administration of prophylaxis before cord-clamping and prophylaxis afterward are also few. Gordon et al.[31] found similar rates of postoperative infection whether they administered prophylactic ampicillin before or after cord-clamping. The review by Swartz and Grolle[25] of 26 studies also showed that antibiotic prophylaxis before operation was as effective as prophylaxis afterward.

As an alternative to parenteral administration of prophylactic antibiotics, Long et al.[32] and Rudd et al.[33] reported excellent results with intraoperative irrigation of the uterus and peritoneal cavity with an antibiotic solution. The potential advantages of this route include decreased cost and, perhaps, decreased toxicity.

However, our group[34] found that there is appreciable absorption of cephalothin, cefamandole, and ampicillin when administered by irrigation. Although the levels were far below that achieved by intravenous administration, the concentrations exceeded the minimal inhibitory concentrations for many genital tract pathogens and were certainly high enough to elicit allergic reactions. Further evaluations of intraoperative irrigation in other populations should prove valuable.

Questions and Adverse Effects

With the use of prophylaxis in cesarean delivery, two special questions arise: Are serious infections decreased, and are there neonatal effects? Although prophylaxis significantly decreases infection, nearly all of these infections are mild and respond promptly to antibiotic therapy. Meade,[35] reviewing 9 series of trials, reported that serious infections (that is, pelvic abscess or septic pelvic thrombophlebitis) occurred in only 0.5% of 659 women receiving prophylaxis and in only 1.1% of 609 controls. In many series no serious infections are reported and no significant decrease (because these complications are so infrequent). Furthermore, in some studies there is no significant decrease in length of hospital stay for patients receiving prophylaxis.[10,13,14,16,20] This finding suggests that postoperative infection in the placebo group does indeed respond promptly.

As to the question about neonatal effects, we concluded that antibiotics administered before cord-clamping rapidly achieved measurable concentrations in the fetus, possibly leading to direct adverse effects or sensitization. More commonly, though, the pediatrician feels impelled to do a sepsis workup and to initiate antibiotic therapy for fear of overlooking a masked sepsis. In view of the equivalent efficacy of prophylaxis administered after cord-clamping, delayed injection would be favored so as to circumvent the problem for the neonate and the pediatrician.

In addition to these concerns, it must also be noted that untoward effects may accompany the use of antibiotics for prophylaxis. These untoward effects include floral changes and direct toxic reactions. Early investigators of prophylaxis made no systematic attempt to identify bacteriologic shifts. With most studies recovering few organisms, there were no apparent shifts toward resistant organisms.

However, investigators in more thorough studies[12,16,23,36] detected significant changes (Table 10–2). In general, there were decreases in highly susceptible organisms and increases in enterococci and Enterobacteriaceae. Although many of the Enterobacteriaceae were susceptible to the prophylactic agent, some unusual resistant isolates such as *Pseudomonas* sp. also appeared. In these cases, the bacterial changes were inconsequential. Nevertheless, it would be unwise to ignore these shifts. When infection develops after prophylaxis, it is essential to obtain appropriate cultures to guide antibiotic therapy. Routine continuation of the agent used for pro-

Table 10–2. Bacteriologic Effects of Prophylactic Antibiotics in Cesarean Section

	Prophylactic Regimen	Effect on Flora of Prophylaxis Group	
Author	(Doses)	Increase	Decrease
Kreutner[12]	Cefazolin (3)	Enterobacteriaceae, *Bacteroides* sp.	Staphylococci, Veillonellaceae, aerobes
Kreutner[16]	Cefamandole or cephalothin (3)	Organisms resistant to prophylactic antibiotics	——
Gibbs[23]	Cefamandole (3)	Enterobacteriaceae, enterococci	Gram-positive anaerobes; nonpathogens
Gibbs[36]	Clindamycin, gentamicin (2)	*Escherichia coli*, enterococci	Anaerobes, aerobic "cocci"

phylaxis may lead to unnecessarily prolonged illness and delayed recognition of the infecting organisms. For the environment, continued widespread use of prophylaxis may produce alarming effects, as Sack[37] has noted recently in regard to the use of antibiotics to prevent "travelers' diarrhea."

Direct toxic effects have been infrequent. Swartz and Grolle[25] noted that in 26 studies no serious allergic or toxic reactions were noted among 1,443 patients receiving prophylaxis. Less serious reactions such as skin rash were occasionally reported. Fatal anaphylactic reactions to prophylactic antibiotics were reported in orthopedic patients,[38] and two cases of fatal pseudomembranous enterocolitis have been attributed to a combination of prophylactic-therapeutic antibiotics.[39]

Alternatives

In view of these adverse effects, it is essential to consider alternatives to routine administration of prophylaxis for obstetric patients. One need is to better delineate target populations for prophylaxis. For example, Gilstrap and Cunningham[6] determined that their patients undergoing cesarean delivery more than 6 hours after membrane rupture ran a risk of postoperative infection as high as 85%. However, other investigators reported the risk to be considerably lower in cesarean section among patients in labor and after membrane rupture. In our patient population,[23] the risk was 54%. However, in predominantly private patients, Harger and English[20] and Polk et al.[21] found the rate of endometritis with primary section to be 20% and 9.4%, respectively. In lower-risk populations, combinations of risk factors may allow determination of target groups, but equations to predict these groups would need to be straightforward.

Examination of amniotic fluid may improve precision in predicting infection. Recent investigations have noted an excellent correlation between positive amniotic fluid cultures collected at cesarean delivery and subsequent postoperative endometritis. Using quantative techniques, Blanco et al.[7] found endometritis in 12 of 13 patients (92%) with $\geq 10^2$ cfu of high-virulence isolate per milliliter soon after delivery.

Among patients with "negative" cultures, endometritis were significantly less common (9 of 23, 39%) ($p < 0.002$). Cooperman et al.[40] reported similar findings with qualitative cultures.

With rapid diagnostic techniques such as gas-liquid chromatography and counterimmunoelectrophoresis of amniotic fluid, it may be possible to identify with great specificity patients in whom endometritis is likely to develop. Thus, in these groups at very high risk, as identified by clinical *and* laboratory techniques, prophylaxis might be used with high efficiency. In groups at considerably lower risk, it may be wiser to treat infection as it becomes clinically evident.

An often-voiced concern about widespread use of prophylaxis is a dangerous relaxation of standard measures to control infection. Hand-washing, appropriate isolation techniques, proper disposal of infected materials and dressings, and changing of soiled scrub suits remain important elements in the control of infections; these precautions cannot be replaced by antibiotic prophylaxis. Iffy et al.[41] noted a decrease in postoperative morbidity from 83% to 16% when these standard infection control measures were strictly enforced. As an important corollary, good intraoperative technique also remains essential. Established principles, including reduction of foreign body, closure of dead space, and avoidance of tissue-crushing and necrosis, must be followed.

As another alternative to prophylaxis, some clinicians have favored early treatment of clinically evident infection. This practice has generally been the norm in low-risk populations.[42] Furthermore, recent reports of excellent cure rates with regimens such as clindamycin-gentamicin and newer penicillins and cephalosporins suggest that it may be better to await clinical evidence of infection even among moderate-risk groups. These therapeutic regimens have resulted in few clinical failures (5%) and few major infection-related complications. The postoperative hospital stay is often brief.[43,44]

Recommendations

For patients undergoing cesarean section, we make the following recommendations:

1. If prophylactic antibiotics for cesarean delivery are used, restrict them to patient groups with a moderate to high risk of postoperative infection.
2. When prophylaxis is used, use a short course of no more than three doses.

3. Select agents for prophylaxis that have been shown to be effective, safe, and inexpensive. For obstetric patients, possible choices are ampicillin and the "first-generation" cephalosporins (including cephalothin and cefazolin).
4. At present, there is no evidence that newer, broad-spectrum β- lactam antibiotics such as cefoxitin, cefamandole, ceftazidime, moxalactam, and piperacillin are more effective as prophylactic agents. In addition, these agents are considerably more expensive.
5. Avoid administration of antibiotic to the fetus by delaying administration until after the cord is clamped.
6. When prophylaxis is used, carefully evaluate patients with postprophylaxis fever or other signs of infection. Perform appropriate cultures. When therapeutic antibiotics are necessary, initially use a broad-spectrum regimen in view of changes in flora brought about by prophylactic antibiotics.

Premature Rupture of the Membranes

Many investigators have used prophylactic antibiotics for either mothers or newborns, but few studies were standardized. Two studies evaluated prophylaxis in infants born after the membranes had been ruptured for 24 hours or more. From a study of 100 such infants, Habel et al.[45] concluded that prophylactic antibiotics were unnecessary because infections were few and that such prophylaxis was hazardous because fungal infections and colonization were increased. On the other hand, Wolf and Olinsky[46] found sepsis in 20% (5 of 25) of cases without prophylaxis. Because there were no cases of sepsis in 24 neonates given penicillin and kanamycin, they recommended prophylaxis until blood culture results were available.

Prophylaxis in mothers with prolonged rupture of the membranes has been more limited than in the past, and is usually reserved for patients undergoing cesarean delivery or those who are undergoing immunosuppression. In the latter setting, Miller et al.[47] in a retrospective study found a decrease (from 18% to 0) in maternal or neonatal infection when prophylactic ampicillin or another antibiotic was used. In another retrospective study, Huff[48] reported a marked decrease in postpartum endometritis in patients with rupture of membranes after 12 hours by using prophylactic penicillin and kanamycin. The decrease was reported for both vaginal and cesarean deliveries.

USES OF PROPHYLAXIS IN GYNECOLOGY

Studies in gynecologic patients have focused mainly on vaginal and abdominal hysterectomy, with some studies of other procedures.

Vaginal Hysterectomy

The risk of postoperative infection in patients undergoing vaginal hysterectomy varies widely. In blind trials of prophylactic antibiotics (Table 10–3) among patients in placebo groups, the proportion with febrile morbidity or diagnosed infection (or both) ranged from 12% to 64%. Since the use of control patients from a comparative study may select patients in high-risk groups, another source is helpful. In the Professional Activity Study,[49] of 3,564 patients having vaginal hysterectomy, 38% had temperatures higher than 101°F. Patients at particularly high risk of infection after vaginal hysterec-

Table 10–3. Double-Blind, Placebo-Controlled, Randomized Studies of Prophylactic Antibiotics in Vaginal Hysterectomy

Author	Antibiotic Regimen (Doses)	No. of Patients	Postoperative Infection Rate[†]	
			Placebo Group (%)	Prophylaxis Group (%)
Forney[50]	Cephaloridine, then cephalexin x 5 days	32	43*	0*
Ledger[51]	Cephaloridine (3)	100	34*	8*
Breeden[52]	Cephaloridine (3)	120	20*	3*
Bivens[53]	Cephalothin, then cephalexin x 6 days	60	20	13
Ohm[54]	Cephaloridine, then cephalexin x 5 days	48	34*	4*
Lett[55]	Cefazolin (1) or cephaloridine (3)	153	61*	14*
Holman[56]	Cefazolin (3)	84	23*	0*
Roberts[57]	Carbenicillin (5)	52	12	0
Mendelson[58]	Cephradine (1 and 4)	66	64*	2*
Grossman[59]	Cefazolin or penicillin x 48 hr	78	25*	6*
Mathews[60]	Trimethoprim-sulfamethoxazole (1)	50	16	8
Polk[61]	Cefazolin (3)	86	21*	2*
Hemsell[62]	Cefoxitin (3)	99	57*	8*
Mickal[63]	Cefoxitin (3)	125	30*	10*

*Significant difference in infection rate, by χ^2 test.

† Infections noted are of the operative site, when information was provided by authors.

tomy are premenopausal women. In another study,[50] there was a higher rate of postoperative infection in women who had hysterectomy within 24 to 72 hours after cervical conization.

A number of double-blind placebo-controlled studies[50-63] showed statistically significant decreases in postoperative infection in patients receiving prophylactic antibiotics (see Table 10–3). Polk[24] reported that the overall preventive fraction was 82% in 11 studies of short-course prophylaxis. Two studies[64,65] evaluated short-course prophylaxis (up to 12 hours) versus long-course prophylaxis (48 to 72 hours). There was no significant difference in infection rates after short-course or long-course prophylaxis in either study.

Three studies compared the efficacy of different antibiotics for prophylaxis. Grossman[59] found no difference between cefazolin and penicillin. Lett[55] reported no significant difference between a single dose of cefazolin and three doses of cephaloridine, and Hamod et al.[65] found cephalothin and metronidazole to be equally effective.

Despite the variety of antibiotics used for prophylaxis, these numerous well-designed studies are remarkably consistent in showing a statistically significant and clinically impressive decrease in postoperative infection. A discussion of side effects and alternatives follows the section on abdominal hysterectomy.

Abdominal Hysterectomy

There has been less interest in antibiotic prophylaxis for abdominal hysterectomy, perhaps because infection after this operation may be less frequent than after vaginal hysterectomy. In four studies[24] evaluating prophylaxis in both kinds of operation, the infection rate was 21% of 136 patients (placebo group) undergoing vaginal hysterectomy and 14% of 367 patients (placebo group) undergoing abdominal hysterectomy. Data from the Professional Activity Study[49] showed that of 8,462 patients who had abdominal hysterectomy, 31% had temperatures higher than 101°F. Infection after abdominal hysterectomy may be less common because of less contamination from the vagina or, perhaps, because of better hemostasis.

Double-blind studies of antibiotic prophylaxis in abdominal hysterectomy are summarized in Table 10–4.[56,57,59,61,66-70] Although not all of these investigators found significant differences, in each study the infection rate was lower in the prophylaxis group. Polk[24]

Table 10–4. Double-Blind, Placebo-Controlled, Randomized Studies of Prophylactic Antibiotics in Abdominal Hysterectomy

Author	Antibiotic Regimen	No. of Patients	Postoperative Infection Rate[†]	
			Placebo Group (%)	Prophylaxis Group (%)
Holman[56]	Cefazolin, 3 doses	80	34*	5*
Roberts[57]	Carbenicillin, 24 hr	47	14	4
Grossman[59]	Cefazolin or penicillin, 48 hr	239	11	8
Polk[61]	Cefazolin, 3 doses	429	13*	7*
Allen[66]	Cephalothin, 5 days	168	30	14
Ohm[67]	Cephaloridine, then cephalexin, 5 days	93	15	6
Mathews[68]	Trimethoprim-sulfamethoxazole	59	38	27
Schepers[69]	Cefoxitin	103	16	6
Duff[70]	Cefoxitin, 2 doses	91	24	18

*Significant difference in infection rate, by χ^2 test.

[†] Infections noted are of the operative site, when information was provided by authors.

reported that in trials of short-course prophylaxis, 49% of postoperative infections were prevented. Only one of these studies compared two agents. In a comparative study[59] of cefazolin and penicillin for prophylaxis, abdominal wound or vaginal cuff infections developed in 5% of 76 patients receiving penicillin and 11% of 79 patients receiving cefazolin. These differences were not significant in these two groups, nor in the placebo group (11% of 84).

Adverse Effects of Prophylaxis in Hysterectomy

Marked changes in flora have been noted in patients receiving 5-day prophylaxis with cephalosporin for both abdominal and vaginal hysterectomy, as well as in patients receiving placebo. Ohm et al.[71,72] noted a shift toward more resistant isolates in patients receiving prophylactic antibiotics. In patients receiving a 48-hour course of prophylaxis, Grossman and Adams[73] reported changes in flora of patients who received short-course prophylaxis for hysterectomy, but these changes were similar to those in patients who received placebo.

Other adverse effects have been reported infrequently. Rashes and abnormalities in screening studies occur rarely. One group of investigators[67] noted difficulty in identifying the source of fever after prophylaxis for 5 days.

Alternative to Prophylaxis in Hysterectomy

In a retrospective study, Richardson et al.,[74] using a nontraumatic technique, reported a decrease in postoperative morbidity and in length of hospital stay. They avoided crushing tissue, heavy suture material, intraabdominal packs, and Foley catheters. The results of application of these fundamental surgical principles are encouraging, but similar prospective studies have not been reported.

Another approach in attempting to decrease the rate of postoperative infection is special preparation of the lower genital tract. Immediately before vaginal hysterectomy, Osborne et al.[75] performed hot conization of the cervix to eliminate the endocervical glands as a contaminable site and then performed a scrub of the vagina and perineum with an iodophore. In their retrospective study, they reported that this preparation was as effective as antibiotic prophylaxis in reducing postoperative infection.

Swartz and Tanaree[76] found a significant decrease in infection after hysterectomy by suction drainage as another alternative. Temperatures higher than 100.4°F developed in 26% of the control patients but in only 11% of patients who had suction drainage. Pelvic infections were decreased from 7% of 100 control patients to none of 100 patients who had suction drainage. In patients who underwent vaginal hysterectomy, temperatures higher than 100.4°F were recorded in 32% of 50 control patients and in 8% of 50 patients with suction drainage; there were 12 pelvic infections (24%) in the control group and only 2 (4%) in the drainage group. Further study[77] showed no further significant difference in postoperative infection when antibiotic prophylaxis was combined with suction drainage.

Recommendations for Vaginal Hysterectomy

1. In premenopausal women and other groups at demonstrably high risk of postoperative infection, prophylactic antibiotics are indicated because they decrease the frequency and the severity of these infections.

2. A short course of prophylaxis involving no more than three doses should be used.
3. Agents that are reasonable choices are the older cephalosporins, penicillin, ampicillin, or tetracycline. Ampicillin and tetracycline have been reported to be effective in nonblind studies.
4. Although they are effective, newer agents have not yet been found to be superior, and they are more expensive.
5. Strict adherence to good surgical technique should not be compromised.

Recommendations for Abdominal Hysterectomy

1. The effectiveness of prophylaxis varies widely from institution to institution, perhaps depending on background infection rates and definitions of infections.
2. Antibiotic prophylaxis would be best reserved for patients with a high risk of pelvic or abdominal wound infection.
3. In these circumstances, the recommendations are the same as for vaginal hysterectomy.

Other Pelvic Surgery

Antibiotic prophylaxis is widely used in major surgery for gynecologic cancer, but randomized trials have been extremely limited. In a double-blind study, Creasman et al.[78] reported that cefamandole significantly reduced pelvic or abdominal infection (from 36% to 4%; $p < 0.01$) in patients having extended hysterectomy for endometrial cancer.

Although Hodgson et al.[79] reported that prophylactic tetracycline decreased complications after first-trimester abortion, the overall infection rate was low, and nearly all of them were "minor" or "minimal." In a double-blind study, Sonne-Holm et al.[80] noted that prophylaxis for this procedure was effective only in patients with previous pelvic inflammatory disease. Thus, except in groups at truly high risk of infection after first-trimester abortion, it would seem much wiser to treat infection as it develops rather than using wide-scale prophylaxis.

REFERENCES

1. PETITTI D, OLSON RO, WILLIAMS RL: Cesarean section in California: 1960 through 1975. Am J Obstet Gynecol 1979;133:391.
2. PLACEK PJ, TAFFEL SM: Trends in cesarean section rates for the United States, 1970-1978. Washington, DC: Public Health Reports 1980;95:540.
3. NIH CONSENSUS DEVELOPMENT TASK FORCE statement on cesarean childbirth. Am J Obstet Gynecol 1981;139:902.
4. GIBBS RS: Clinical risk factors for puerperal infection. Obstet Gynecol 1980;55:178S.
5. GIBBS RS, JONES PM, WILDER CJY: Internal fetal monitoring and maternal infection following cesarean section: A prospective study. Obstet Gynecol 1978;52:193.
6. GILSTRAP LC III, CUNNINGHAM FG: The bacterial pathogenesis of infection following cesarean section. Obstet Gynecol 1979;53:545.
7. BLANCO JD, GIBBS RS, CASTANEDA YS et al: Correlation of quantitative amniotic fluid cultures with endometritis after cesarean section. Am J Obstet Gynecol 1982;143:897.
8. GIBBS RS, DeCHERNEY AM, SCHWARZ RH: Prophylactic antibiotics in cesarean section: A double-blind study. Am J Obstet Gynecol 1972;114:1048.
9. GIBBS RS, HUNT JE, SCHWARZ RH: A follow-up study on prophylactic antibiotics in cesarean section. Am J Obstet Gynecol 1973;117:419.
10. WORK BA Jr: Role of preventive antibiotics in patients undergoing cesarean section. South Med J 1979;70,Suppl 1:44.
11. WONG R, GEE CL, LEDGER WJ: Prophylactic use of cefazolin in monitored obstetric patients undergoing cesarean section. Obstet Gynecol 1978;51:407.
12. KREUTNER AK, DEL BENE VE, DELAMAR D et al: Perioperative antibiotic prophylaxis in cesarean section. Obstet Gynecol 1978;52:279.
13. GALL SA: The efficacy of prophylactic antibiotics in cesarean section. Am J Obstet Gynecol 1979;134:506.
14. PHELAN JP, PRUYN SC: Prophylactic antibiotics in cesarean section: A double-blind study of cefazolin. Am J Obstet Gynecol 1979;133:474.
15. LARSON P, NELSON KE, ISMAIL M et al: Double-blind study of cefoxitin prophylaxis of post-cesarean section infection. *In:*

Current Chemotherapy and Infectious Disease: Proceedings of the 11th International Congress of Chemotherapy and the 19th Interscience Conference on Antimicrobial Agents and Chemotherapy. Washington, DC: American Society of Microbiology; 1980:1212–1214.

16. KREUTNER AK, DEL BENE VE, DELAMAR D et al: Perioperative cephalosporin prophylaxis in cesarean section: Effect on endometritis in the high-risk patient. Am J Obstet Gynecol 1979;134:925.

17. DUFF P, PARK RC: Antibiotic prophylaxis for cesarean section in a military population. Milit Med 1980;145:377.

18. McCOWAN L, JACKSON P: The prophylactic use of metronidazole in Ceasarean section. NZ Med J 1980;92:153.

19. REHU M, JAHKOLA M: Prophylactic antibiotics in cesarean section: Effect of a short preoperative course of benzyl penicillin or clindamycin plus gentamicin on postoperative infectious morbidity. Ann Clin Res 1980;12:45.

20. HARGER JH, ENGLISH DH: Selection of patients for antibiotic prophylaxis in cesarean sections. Am J Obstet Gynecol 1981;141:752.

21. POLK BF, KRACHE M, PHILLIPPE M et al: Randomized clinical trial of perioperative cefoxitin in preventing maternal infection after primary cesarean section. Am J Obstet Gynecol 1982;142:983.

22. DILLON WP, SEIGEL MS, LELE AS et al: Evaluation of cefoxitin prophylaxis for cesarean section. Int J Obstet Gynaecol 1981;19:133.

23. GIBBS RS, St CLAIR PJ, CASTILLO MS et al: Bacteriologic effects of antibiotic prophylaxis in high-risk cesarean section. Obstet Gynecol 1981;57:277.

24. POLK BF: Antimicrobial prophylaxis to prevent mixed bacterial infection. J Antimicrob Chemother 1981;8, Suppl D:115.

25. SWARTZ WH, GROLLE K: The use of prophylactic antibiotics in cesarean section: A review of the literature. J Reprod Med 1981;26:595.

26. ITSKOVITZ J, PALDI E, KATZ M: The effect of prophylactic antibiotics on febrile morbidity following cesarean section. Obstet Gynecol 1979;53:162.

27. VAUGHN JE: Comparison of metronidazole and cephradine in the prevention of wound sepsis following Caesarean section. In: Royal Society of Medicine International Congress and Symposium Series, No 18;1979:203.

28. STIVER HG, FORWARD KR, LIVINGSTONE RA et al: Multicenter comparison of cefoxitin versus cefazolin for prevention of infectious morbidity after nonelective cesarean section. Am J Obstet Gynecol 1983;145:158.

29. D'ANGELO LJ, SOKOL RJ: Short- versus long-course prophylactic antibiotic treatment in cesarean section patients. Obstet Gynecol 1980;55:583.

30. AYANGADE O: Long- vs short-course antibiotic prophylaxis in cesarean section: A comparative clinical study. J Natl Med Assoc 1979;71:71.

31. GORDON HR, PHELPS D, BLANCHARD K: Prophylactic cesarean section antibiotics: Maternal and neonatal morbidity before or after cord clamping. Obstet Gynecol 1979;53:151.

32. LONG WH, RUDD EG, DILLON MB: Intrauterine irrigation with cefamandole nafate solution at cesarean section: A preliminary report. Am J Obstet Gynecol 1980;138:755.

33. RUDD EG, COBEY EA, LONG WH et al: Prevention of endomyometritis using antibiotic irrigation during cesarean section. Obstet Gynecol 1982;60:413.

34. DUFF P, GIBBS RS, JORGENSEN JH et al: The pharmacokinetics of prophylactic antibiotics administered by intraoperative irrigation at the time of cesarean section. Obstet Gynecol 1982;60:409.

35. MEAD PB: Prophylactic antibiotics and antibiotic resistance. Semin Perinatol 1977;1:101.

36. GIBBS RS, WEINSTEIN AJ: Bacteriologic effects of prophylactic antibiotics in cesarean section. Am J Obstet Gynecol 1976;126:226.

37. SACK RB: Prophylactic antibiotics? The individual versus the community. N Engl J Med 1979;300:1107 (Editorial).

38. SPRUILL FG, MINETTE LJ, STURNER WQ: Two surgical deaths associated with cephalothin. JAMA 1974;229:440.

39. LEDGER WJ, PUTTLER OL: Death from pseudomembranous enterocolitis. Obstet Gynecol 1975;45:609.

40. COOPERMAN NR, KASIM M, RAJASHEKARAIAH KR: Clinical significance of amniotic fluid, amniotic membranes, and endometrial biopsy cultures at the time of cesarean section. Am J Obstet Gynecol 1980;137:536.

41. IFFY L, KAMINETZKY HA, MAIDMAN JE et al: Control of perinatal infection by traditional preventive measures. Obstet Gynecol 1979;54:403.

42. Prophylactic antibiotics in caesarean section. Br Med J 1973; 1:675.

43. DiZEREGA G, YONEKURA L, ROY S et al: A comparison of clindamycin-gentamicin and penicillin-gentamicin in the treatment of post-cesarean section endomyometritis. Am J Obstet Gynecol 1979;134:238.

44. GIBBS RS, BLANCO JD, CASTANEDA YS et al: A double-blind, randomized comparison of clindamycin-gentamicin versus cefamandole for treatment of post-cesarean section endomyometritis. Am J Obstet Gynecol 1982;144:261.

45. HABEL AH, SANDOR GS, CONN NK et al: Premature rupture of membranes and effects of prophylactic antibiotics. Arch Dis Child 1972;47:401.

46. WOLF RL, OLINSKY A: Prolonged rupture of fetal membranes and neonatal infections. S Afr Med J 1976;50:574.

47. MILLER JM Jr, BRAZY JE, GALL SA et al: Premature rupture of the membranes: Maternal and neonatal infectious morbidity related to betamethasone and antibiotic therapy. J Reprod Med 1980;25:173.

48. HUFF RW: Antibiotic prophylaxis for puerperal endometritis following premature rupture of the membranes. J Reprod Med 1977;19:79.

49. LEDGER WJ, CHILD MA: The hospital care of patients undergoing hysterectomy: An analysis of 12,026 patients from the Professional Activity Study. Am J Obstet Gynecol 1973; 117:423.

50. FORNEY JP, MORROW CP, TOWNSEND DE et al: Impact of cephalosporin prophylaxis on conization: Vaginal hysterectomy morbidity. Am J Obstet Gynecol 1976;125:100.

51. LEDGER WJ, SWEET RL, HEADINGTON JT: Prophylactic cephaloridine in the prevention of postoperative pelvic infections in premenopausal women undergoing vaginal hysterectomy. Am J Obstet Gynecol 1973;115:766.

52. BREEDEN JT, MAYO JE: Low dose prophylactic antibiotics in vaginal hysterectomy. Obstet Gynecol 1974;43:379.

53. BIVENS MD, NEUFELD J, McCARTY WD: The prophylactic use of Keflex and Keflin in vaginal hysterectomy. Am J Obstet Gynecol 1975;122:169.

54. OHM MJ, GALASK RP: The effect of antibiotic prophylaxis on patients undergoing vaginal operations. I. The effect on morbidity. Am J Obstet Gynecol 1975;123:590.

55. LETT WJ, ANSBACHER R, DAVISON BL et al: Prophylactic antibiotics for women undergoing vaginal hysterectomy. J Reprod Med 1977;19:51.

56. HOLMAN JF, McGOWAN JE, THOMPSON JD: Perioperative antibiotics in major elective gynecologic surgery. South Med J 1978;71:417.

57. ROBERTS JM, HOMESLEY HD: Low-dose carbenicillin prophylaxis for vaginal and abdominal hysterectomy. Obstet Gynecol 1978;52:83.

58. MENDELSON J, PORTNOY J, DE SAINT VICTOR JR et al: Effect of single and multidose cephradine prophylaxis on infectious morbidity of vaginal hysterectomy. Obstet Gynecol 1979; 53:31.

59. GROSSMAN JH III, GRECO TP, MINKIN MJ et al: Prophylactic antibiotics in gynecologic surgery. Obstet Gynecol 1979; 53:537.

60. MATHEWS DD, AGARWAL V, GORDON AM et al: A double-blind trial of single-dose chemoprophylaxis with co-trimoxazole during vaginal hysterectomy and repair. Br J Obstet Gynaecol 1979;86:737.

61. POLK BF, TAGER IB, SHAPIRO M et al: Randomised clinical trial of perioperative cefazolin in preventing infection after hysterectomy. Lancet 1980;1:437.

62. HEMSELL DL, CUNNINGHAM FG, KAPPUS S et al: Cefoxitin for prophylaxis in premenopausal women undergoing vaginal hysterectomy. Obstet Gynecol 1980;56:629.

63. MICKAL A, CUROLE D, LEWIS C: Cefoxitin sodium: Double-blind vaginal hysterectomy prophylaxis in premenopausal patients. Obstet Gynecol 1980;56:222.

64. LEDGER WJ, GEE C, LEWIS WP: Guidelines for antibiotic prophylaxis in gynecology. Am J Obstet Gynecol 1975; 121:1038.

65. HAMOD KA, SPENCE MR, ROSENSHEIN NB et al: Single-dose and multidose prophylaxis in vaginal hysterectomy: A comparison of sodium cephalothin and metronidazole. Am J Obstet Gynecol 1980;136:976.

66. ALLEN JL, RAMPONE JF, WHEELESS CR: Use of a prophylactic antibiotic in elective major gynecologic operations. Obstet Gynecol 1972;39:218.

67. OHM MJ, GALASK RP: The effect of antibiotic prophylaxis on patients undergoing total abdominal hysterectomy. I. Effect on morbidity. Am J Obstet Gynecol 1976;125:442.

68. MATHEWS DD, ROSS H, COOPER J: A double-blind trial of single-dose chemoprophylaxis with co-trimoxazole during total abdominal hysterectomy. Br J Obstet Gynaecol 1977; 84:894.

69. SCHEPERS JP, MERKUS FWHM: Cefoxitin sodium: Double-blind, placebo-controlled, prophylactic study in premenopausal patients undergoing abdominal hysterectomy. Clin Pharmacol Ther 1981;29:281 (Abstract).

70. DUFF P: Antibiotic prophylaxis for abdominal hysterectomy. Obstet Gynecol 1982;60:25.

71. OHM MJ, GALASK RP: The effect of antibiotic prophylaxis on patients undergoing vaginal operations. II. Alterations of microbial flora. Am J Obstet Gynecol 1975;123:597.

72. OHM MJ, GALASK RP: The effect of antibiotic prophylaxis on patients undergoing total abdominal hysterectomy. II. Alterations of microbial flora. Am J Obstet Gynecol 1976;125:448.

73. GROSSMAN JH III, ADAMS RL: Vaginal flora in women undergoing hysterectomy with antibiotic prophylaxis. Obstet Gynecol 1979;53:23.

74. RICHARDSON AC, LYON JB, GRAHAM EE: Abdominal hysterectomy: Relationship between morbidity and surgical technique. Am J Obstet Gynecol 1973;115:953.

75. OSBORNE NG, WRIGHT RC, DUBAY M: Preoperative hot conization of the cervix: A possible method to reduce postoperative febrile morbidity following vaginal hysterectomy. Am J Obstet Gynecol 1979;133:374.

76. SWARTZ WH, TANAREE P: Suction drainage as an alternative to prophylactic antibiotics for hysterectomy. Obstet Gynecol 1975;45:305.

77. SWARTZ WH, TANAREE P: T-tube suction drainage and/or prophylactic antibiotics: A randomized study of 451 hysterectomies. Obstet Gynecol 1976;47:665.

78. CREASMAN WT, HILL GB, WEED JC Jr et al: A trial of prophylactic cefamandole in extended gynecologic surgery. Obstet Gynecol 1982;59:309.

79. HODGSON JE, MAJOR B, PORTMANN K et al: Prophylactic use of tetracycline for first trimester abortions. Obstet Gynecol 1975;45:574.

80. SONNE-HOLM S, HEISTERBERG L, HEBJØRN S et al: Prophylactic antibiotics in first-trimester abortions: A clinical, controlled trial. Am J Obstet Gynecol 1981;139:693.

Appendix

GUIDELINE FOR PREVENTION OF SURGICAL WOUND INFECTIONS

Bryan P. Simmons, M.D.

WORKING GROUP

J. Wesley Alexander, M.D.
Professor of Surgery
Director of Transplantation
University of Cincinnati Medical Center
Director of Research
Shriners' Burn Institute
Cincinnati, Ohio

N. Joel Ehrenkranz, M.D.
Director, South Florida Hospital Consortium for Infection Control
Miami, Florida

Robert H. Fitzgerald, Jr., M.D.
Associate Professor of Orthopedic Surgery
Consultant, Orthopedic Surgery
Mayo Clinic
Rochester, Minnesota

Allen B. Kaiser, M.D.
Chief, Department of Medicine
Hospital Epidemiologist
St. Thomas Hospital
Associate Professor of Medicine
Vanderbilt University School of Medicine
Nashville, Tennessee

From Infection Control 1982;3:188-196, with the permission of the U.S. Centers for Disease Control. The Guideline was written by Bryan P. Simmons, M.D.

William J. Ledger, M.D.
Given Foundation Professor of Obstetrics and Gynecology
Cornell University Medical Center
Obstetrician and Gynecologist-in-Chief
The New York Hospital
New York, New York

Jonathan L. Meakins, Jr., M.D.
Associate Professor of Surgery and Microbiology
McGill University
Montreal, Canada

Colonel Darlene K. McLeod, ANC
Nursing Consultant
Office of the Surgeon General
U.S. Army
Washington, D.C.

Hiram C. Polk, Jr., M.D.
Professor and Chairman
Department of Surgery
University of Louisville School of Medicine
Louisville, Kentucky

INTRODUCTION

Patients who undergo a surgical operation are at high risk of having one or more nosocomial infections. These infections develop in more surgical patients (8%) than in any other patient group, and about 70% of all nosocomial infections throughout the hospital develop in patients who have an operation.[1] Most infections in surgical patients, however, are not related to the wound but to instrumentation of the urinary and respiratory tracts. Thus, personnel who take care of these patients should be aware of measures to prevent nosocomial infections at all sites. Moreover, to prevent surgical wound infections, personnel who perform the operation must take the lead in instituting prevention measures, because the most important measures involve use of good surgical technique and are not easily instituted simply by making changes in hospital policy.

Surgical wound infections are the second most frequent nosocomial infection and are an important cause of increased costs, morbidity, and death for patients. They are divided into infections related to 1) the incisional wound and 2) structures adjacent to the wound that were entered or exposed during an operation (sometimes called "deep infections"). Some 60%–80% of infections are incisional, and the rest are at adjacent sites, for example, intraabdominal/retroperitoneal and deep soft tissue.[1,2] This guideline deals primarily with incisional infections, although many recommendations in it will also help prevent other surgical wound infections. Burn wounds are not discussed.

EPIDEMIOLOGY

In general, a wound can be considered infected if purulent material drains from it, even if a culture is negative or not taken.[3] This definition has advantages when compared with those based on culture results because 1) a positive culture does not necessarily indicate infection, since many wounds, infected or not, are colonized by bacteria, and 2) infected wounds may not yield pathogens by culture because the pathogens are fastidious, culture techniques are inadequate, or the patient has been treated. Because infections occur in a variety of ways and may not always produce significant purulent material, it is also useful to consider a wound infected (but not to consider a purulent wound uninfected) if the attending physician believes it to be. Unless the incision is involved, stitch abscesses probably should not be considered infected wounds, but should be monitored and listed separately from other infections.

Wounds can be classified according to the likelihood and degree of wound contamination at the time of operation. A widely accepted classification scheme[3-5] is listed below:

Clean Wounds

These are uninfected operative wounds in which no inflammation is encountered, and neither the respiratory, alimentary, or genitourinary tract nor the oropharyngeal cavity is entered. In addition, they are elective, primarily closed, and if necessary, drained with closed drainage. Operative incisional wounds that follow nonpenetrating (blunt) trauma should be included in this category if they meet the criteria.

Clean-Contaminated Wounds

These are operative wounds in which the respiratory, aliment-ary, or genitourinary tract is entered under controlled conditions and without unusual contamination. Specifically, operations involving the biliary tract, appendix, vagina, and oropharynx are included in this category, provided no evidence of infection or major break in technique is encountered.

Contaminated Wounds

These include open, fresh, accidental wounds, operations with major breaks in sterile technique or gross spillage from the gas-trointestinal tract, and incisions in which acute, nonpurulent inflammation is encountered.

Dirty and Infected Wounds

These include old traumatic wounds with retained devitalized tissue and those that involve existing clinical infection or per-forated viscera. This definition suggests that the organisms causing postoperative infection were present in the operative field before operation.

This classification scheme has been shown in numerous studies to predict the relative probability that a wound will become infected. Clean wounds have a 1%–5% risk of infection; clean contaminated, 8%–11%; contaminated, 15%–17%; and dirty, over 27%.[3,6] These infection rates were affected by many appropriate prevention measures taken during the studies, such as use of prophylactic antibiotics, and would have been higher if no prevention measures had been taken. In addition to its application to predicting the probability of infection, this classification has other uses. By stan-dardizing many important factors other than surgical technique, it often allows valid comparison of wound infection rates associated with different techniques, surgeons, hospitals, etc. This comparison is useful for research and for increasing awareness of surgical wound infections. For a given operation, the clean-wound infection rate, in particular, can be so standardized that it can be used by surgeons to compare their own infection rate, and by inference, technique, with that of other surgeons.[6] The classification also serves to alert personnel to wounds at high risk of infection, for example, dirty wounds, and thus enable personnel to take appropriate preventive and surveillance measures.

Although the degree of operative contamination of wounds is important in determining the risk of infection, so are many host and local wound factors. The host factors leading to increased risk may include very young or old age, marked obesity, presence of a perioperative infection, use of steroids (glucocorticoid), and, possibly, diabetes and severe malnutrition.[3] Local wound factors associated with high risk include presence of devitalized tissue or foreign bodies and poor blood supply to the wound. The location of the wound can also affect the likelihood of infection; wounds located in areas that are easily contaminated, for example, near the anus, are more frequently infected.

Surgical wound infections are usually localized to the wound and do not, with appropriate treatment, result in major complications. However, infection can result in several kinds of severe local and systemic complications. Local ones include destruction of tissue and separation of the wound, failure of the operation, incisional and deep hernias, septic thrombophlebitis, recurrent pain, and disfiguring and disabling scars. Systemic complications are numerous and include fever; increased metabolic demands that sometimes result in malnutrition; bacteremia; shock; metastatic infection; failure of vital organs remote from the infection; and death. The frequency and severity of each complication depends in large part on the infecting pathogen and on the site of infection. For example, *Streptococcus viridans* is unlikely to cause a severe infection unless it invades the vascular system, whereas a group A streptococcal infection is likely to be severe regardless of the site. Further, any infection involving an implanted foreign body or substantial necrotic tissue is likely to have serious sequelae regardless of the pathogen involved.

As determined by reports to the National Nosocomial Infection Study (NNIS), gram-negative bacteria (as a group) make up the majority of pathogens isolated from surgical wounds. However, *Staphylococcus aureus* is the most frequently isolated single pathogen. Pathogens other than bacteria, for example, fungi and viruses, are uncommonly reported. Pathogens that are likely to be isolated vary, depending on the operation, institution, the occurrence of epidemics, and other pertinent factors.

Pathogens that infect surgical wounds can be acquired from the patient, that is, an endogenous source, or from the hospital environment or personnel, that is, an exogenous source. Endogenous sources appear to be responsible for most infections, especially if clean-wound infections are excluded.[3,4] Sources of endogenous contamination include the gastrointestinal and genitourinary tracts, sites of active infection remote from the wound (for example, a urinary tract infection is often a remote infection), the skin, and anterior nares.

Exogenous contamination is responsible for a substantial proportion of infections in clean wounds. During epidemic periods, exogenous contamination may be responsible for many more infections. A recent publication lists many microorganisms reported to cause epidemics of surgical wound infections and the likely source of these microorganisms.[7] Exogenous contamination may come from any personnel or environmental source, although direct contact with the wound by the surgical team is probably the final pathway for spread of such contamination. Epidemics of infections due to *S. aureus* and group A *Streptococcus* suggest personnel carriers as a source. Epidemics due to gram-negative microorganisms may be spread from environmental sources, especially those containing water (for example, irrigating solutions) and anesthesia and respiratory therapy equipment. Most infections, endogenous or exogenous, appear to result from contamination acquired in the operating room. Few infections are acquired after the operation if wounds are closed primarily, that is, before leaving the operating room, and drains are not used, probably because the normal healing process seals most wounds within hours after closure.

CONTROL MEASURES

The risk of developing a surgical wound infection is largely determined by three factors:

1. the amount and type of microbial contamination of the wound,
2. the condition of the wound at the end of the operation (largely determined by surgical technique and disease processes encountered during the operation), and
3. host susceptibility, that is, the patient's intrinsic ability to deal with microbial contamination.

These factors interact in a complex manner. For example, a wound in healthy tissue is surprisingly resistant to infection even when contaminated with many microorganisms, whereas a wound containing foreign or necrotic material is highly susceptible to infection even if few microorganisms are present. Measures intended to prevent surgical wound infections are directed at all three factors just mentioned, but especially the first two. Since most infections are acquired in the operating room and good surgical practices are crucial to their prevention, most prevention measures should be directed at influencing the practices of the surgical team.

Measures aimed at preventing microbial contamination of the wound begin before the operation does. One important preoperative and postoperative measure is to treat active infections. Patients who have an active bacterial infection, even if it is at a site remote from the surgical wound, have a much greater risk of wound infection than do uninfected patients.[3] Treating a "remote" infection that is present before or after an operation is believed to reduce the risk of wound infection.

Other preoperative measures involving the patient are these: keeping the preoperative hospital stay short, bathing with antiseptics, avoiding hair removal or, if necessary, removing hair with clippers or depilatories rather than a razor, and preparing the operative site with an antiseptic. A short preoperative stay has been associated with low wound infection rates;[1,3,6,8] this finding may result from reduced colonization of surgical patients with nosocomial pathogens that can later contaminate the wound. It has been suggested that limiting the preoperative stay to the minimum time necessary may reduce the risk of infection,[6] but there are no adequate data to support this practice. Bathing by the patient with antiseptics has been recommended as a preoperative prevention measure because it reduces colonization with typical wound pathogens such as *S. aureus*.[8] Although such bathing is easy, safe, and inexpensive, it has not been proven to reduce infections. Hair adjacent to the operative site is often removed to prevent the wound from becoming contaminated with hair during the operation. However, hair removal can injure the skin, and such injury may increase the risk of infection[6,9] by promoting increased skin colonization with bacteria. Using clippers or a depilatory to remove hair seems to cause less skin injury than using a razor. If hair removal is necessary, doing it immediately before the operation may reduce the risk of infection.[9]

To reduce further the risk of contaminating the wound with a patient's own microorganisms, antiseptic agents are used to prepare the skin at the operative site before the operation. First, the site is thoroughly scrubbed with a detergent solution to remove superficial flora, soil, and debris that could interfere with antisepsis. Immediately before the operation, an antiseptic solution is applied to kill or inhibit more adherent, deep, resident flora. Many antiseptics (see Guidelines for Hospital Environmental Control: Antiseptics, Handwashing, and Handwashing Facilities) have been used to prepare the operative site, but tincture of chlorhexidine or iodophors offer several advantages over the others. Both have an excellent spectrum of activity against bacteria. Tincture of chlorhexidine has rapid and persistent antibacterial activity. Iodophors also act rapidly and have persistent activity if they are not wiped off. Tincture of iodine is also an excellent surgical prepping agent but can cause skin burns, although this is unusual with a 1% tincture. Alcohol acts rapidly but has no persistent effect after it evaporates. Hexachlorophene has been used as a preoperative skin prep, but it has poor activity against gram-negative organisms and requires repeated use for maximum effectiveness. In addition, hexachlorophene can be absorbed from the skin and in large amounts might have toxic effects on the central nervous system, particularly in premature infants.

The surgical team must also take perioperative measures to prevent microbial contamination of the wound. Contamination from the surgical team may result from direct contact, usually with hands, or from contaminated air, usually the result of shedding from skin or mucous membranes. Transfer of microorganisms from hands to the wound is reduced by scrubbing the hands and using sterile gloves. The surgical scrub is designed to kill or remove as many bacteria as possible, including resident bacteria. Maximal elimination of bacteria requires use of antiseptics and careful scrubbing; removing hand jewelry and cleaning around the nails is important because jewelry and nails can harbor bacteria. Chlorhexidine, iodophors, and hexachlorophene can be used for the preoperative hand scrub; however, hexachlorophene must be used consistently and frequently (for example, several times a day) if it is to be maximally effective. The ideal duration of the surgical scrub is not known, but times as short as five minutes appear safe.[10,11] Once hands are scrubbed, sterile gloves act as an additional barrier to bacterial transfer to the wound (in addition to protecting the wearer from microorganisms infecting the patient). Bacteria can multiply rapidly under gloves and can contaminate the wound through punctures in gloves, which occur frequently;[12] use of antiseptics for handwashing before gloving will retard bacterial growth.

Air is also a potential source of microorganisms that can contaminate surgical wounds; its role in wound infections has been demonstrated in certain clean operations,[3] such as operations in which a foreign body is implanted. Operating room (OR) air is often contaminated with microorganisms that are usually attached to other airborne particles such as dust, lint, skin squames, or respiratory droplets. Many of these microorganisms are "pathogens" by usual definitions. The number of viable airborne microorganisms for a given amount of OR ventilation is largely proportional to human activity. Greater numbers of airborne microorganisms can be expected with increased numbers of persons, especially if the persons are moving or have uncovered skin areas. Airborne contamination decreases with

1. decreased numbers and activity of personnel,
2. increased ventilation that dilutes contaminated air with relatively clean filtered or outdoor air,
3. ultraviolet light, which kills microorganisms, and
4. occlusive clothing, masks, and gloves, which reduce shedding into air.

Movement or activity in the OR can be decreased by closing the OR door and by limiting the number of personnel in the OR and adjacent corridors. In addition to limiting unnecessary activity, closing the door will decrease mixing of the OR air with corridor air, which usually contains relatively high counts of bacteria. Limiting personnel movement in the OR and adjacent corridors takes planning. The goal of such planning, often called "traffic control," is to make ORs self-sufficient, or nearly so, once an operation has begun.

To reduce airborne contamination, some researchers recommend "laminar flow" ventilation units for use in ORs, especially for those rooms used for surgical placement of implants, because these ventilation units provide highly clean and nearly sterile air with minimal air turbulence. However, the ventilation recommended for modern ORs, 15 to 25 changes of highly filtered air per hour depending on the amount of fresh air,[13] appears to be adequate to remove most airborne microorganisms.[14] In addition, laminar flow units are very expensive, and although currently under study, they have not been subjected to an adequate trial of their efficacy (or cost-effectiveness) in preventing infections.

Like laminar flow systems, ultraviolet (UV) irradiation provides an atmosphere free of most viable bacteria. UV-irradiated operating rooms have been shown to produce a small but statistically significant decrease in infections of clean surgical wounds, although infections of all surgical wounds combined were not reduced.[3] UV requires routine use of a visor or goggles and skin protection to prevent burns. UV lights require frequent, routine maintenance to monitor the intensity of UV light and for cleaning.

Microorganisms are constantly being shed from exposed skin and mucous membranes, so masks, drapes, hoods, and gowns are used as barriers to decrease shedding into the air and prevent wound contamination. These barriers are most effective when their pore size is so small that they do not allow passage of bacteria, even during use and when wet. Several woven and nonwoven fabrics are virtually impermeable to bacteria.[15] When drapes and gowns made from such material were used in a recent study, a reduction in wound infections occurred.[16] Gowns made of tightly woven cotton treated with a water repellent are reusable and prevent passage of bacteria, provided they have not been laundered and sterilized more than 75 times.[17] (Some hospitals mark these gowns with an expiration date that is determined by the usual time it takes for gowns to be laundered 75 times.) Some gowns are made entirely of impermeable materials while others have these materials in key areas, such as in the front and on the sleeves. These materials are most effective if they cover virtually all exposed skin (and hair) surfaces of the team and the patient. However, team members may get uncomfortably hot in gowns made only of these materials unless the room temperature is lowered or ventilation is increased. Some surgeons use a separate ventilation (aspirator) system inside a helmet and gown to remove air. Such systems not only cool the surgeon but remove microorganisms as they are shed inside the helmet and gown.

In the modern, well-managed OR, the risk of infection related to the inanimate environment appears low. This is due, in great part, to adequate sterilization of surgical devices (see Guidelines for Hospital Environmental Control: Cleaning, Disinfection, and Sterilization of Hospital Equipment), ventilation systems that provide clean air, and adequate cleaning of the OR. If sound routine cleaning methods[5,18] are strictly enforced and OR ventilation is adequate, the OR should be adequately clean, and environmental culturing and special cleaning after "dirty" cases should not be useful. Some architectural designs incorporated into ORs may be useful in maintaining a clean environment.[19] Others, however, such as floor plans that use a central clean area and a peripheral traffic corridor, have not been proven to be especially useful. In addition, tacky or antiseptic mats placed at the entrance to OR suites to prevent contamination from entering with personnel can be a nuisance and have not been shown to reduce the risk of infection.

The most important measure to prevent wound infections is using good operative technique. Poor technique can result in inadvertent contamination of the wound (for example, as may occur with accidental perforation of the bowel during an abdominal operation), may prolong the operation, and may result in a wound that cannot adequately resist infection because it contains devitalized tissues or inappropriate foreign bodies. Since the risk of wound infection increases with the length of the operation, an expeditious operation is important.[1,3,6] However, the surgeon must balance the need to operate quickly with the need to handle tissues gently, reduce bleeding and hematoma formation, eradicate dead space, and minimize devitalized tissue and foreign materials in the wound. Other prevention techniques are not as well established as those just mentioned but appear prudent to use when possible. These are use of fine and monofilament rather than thick or braided suture and minimal use of suture and cautery. Technique applies not only to a surgeon's skill in handling the wound, but also to skill in supervising the surgical team and maintaining professional decorum that facilitates prompt and successful operations. Poor discipline in the OR can result in mistakes and sloppy aseptic technique. Once a surgeon has finished training, surgical habits might not be easy to alter, but improvement may be stimulated by informing surgeons of their rate of infections in clean wounds.[6]

The postoperative period usually does not contribute greatly to the risk of surgical wound infections. Nevertheless, wounds can become contaminated and later become infected if they are touched by contaminated hands or objects after the operation, especially if the wound is not closed during the operation (primarily closed) or if a drain is used. Until wound edges are sealed and the wound is clearly healing (about 24 hours after operation for most wounds), wounds are covered with sterile dressings to reduce the risk of such contamination. A recently developed, transparent, semipermeable membrane dressing is being promoted for use on wounds because the dressing does not need to be removed for the wound to be observed; the value of using this dressing is unproven. Most dressings are occasionally removed for the wound to be observed and, if necessary, treated; the frequency of removal depends on such factors as the type of wound, the presence of infection, drainage, moisture, pain, fever, and so forth. Personnel taking care of wounds can reduce the risk of contamination by washing their hands and avoiding contact with the wound (the no-touch technique) or, if contact with the wound is necessary, wearing sterile gloves.

In the postoperative period, reducing the risk of wound infection can be facilitated by adequate wound drainage. If not allowed to drain freely, blood, pus, body fluids, and necrotic material collect in a wound and provide a growth medium for microorganisms. Further, pus and microorganisms not allowed to drain may cause bacteremia as pressure in the wound builds. However, if a wound is drained, especially if this is done with open drainage, the skin cannot be completely closed and microorganisms can enter the wound or deeper structures and cause infection. Thus, surgeons routinely drain only wounds expected to produce significant amounts of blood or other drainage and use closed drainage in preference to open (penrose) drainage.[20,21] If a drain is used, having it enter through an adjacent, separate stab wound rather than the primary surgical wound will reduce the risk of infection. For dirty wounds, delaying wound closure is preferable to inserting a drain and reduces the risk of infection;[22] delayed wound closure is also useful for many contaminated wounds.

A patient's intrinsic susceptibility to infection, that is, host susceptibility, is also important in determining the risk of infection. Unlike many other risk factors, host susceptibility is often not easily altered. However, if the operation can be delayed, some host factors can be altered: 1) diabetics can have their blood sugars better controlled, 2) severely obese patients can lose weight, 3) patients on steroids may be able to discontinue them or have the dosage reduced, and 4) severely malnourished patients can receive oral or parenteral hyperalimentation. There is no definitive evidence that these alterations will reduce the risk of infection. In each example and in others in which host susceptibility can be altered, the physician must weigh the benefits of the alteration against the risk of a delayed operation or other factors associated with intervention.

For some operations, prophylactic antibiotics are a means of reducing the risk of wound infections. Prophylaxis, that is, antibiotic administration *before* an infection occurs, is effective probably because it reduces wound contamination to a level that can be handled by the body's immune defenses; this level varies, depending on the condition of the wound and immune defenses. Prophylaxis is most useful for operations associated with a moderate level of contamination (clean-contaminated operations). Prophylaxis is not worthwhile for clean operations unless the consequences of infection are severe or life-threatening, for example, as occurs with prosthetic (implant) orthopedic and vascular surgery. Antibiotics are also used for dirty operations but are for treatment rather than prophylaxis.[4]

Prophylaxis may be administered parenterally or, for intestinal operations, orally. To be most effective, parenteral prophylaxis should be administered shortly before the operation begins so that therapeutic levels of antibiotics are present in the wound during the operation.[23] Continuing parenteral prophylaxis longer than 24 hours increases the risk of antibiotic toxicity and selection of resistant strains of bacteria but does not further reduce the risk of infection.[24] Oral prophylaxis is used primarily for intestinal operations as a bowel preparation. It is best to administer oral prophylaxis for one day before the operation and not continue it afterwards. Parenteral and oral prophylaxis are about equally effective for intestinal operations.[25] Parenteral prophylaxis for prevention of bacterial endocarditis may also be indicated before an operation, but only its use before cardiac operations is addressed in this guideline.

To decrease the risk of infection, surgeons sometimes put antibiotics and antiseptics directly into a wound, often as an irrigation solution.[26] Antibiotics may have a role for local wound care during the operation, although such use has not been adequately compared to the use of parenteral prophylactic antibiotics. Some antibiotics used to irrigate the wound can be absorbed and have systemic toxic effects. Some antiseptics, alcohol, for example, are toxic to tissues other than skin or mucous membranes and should not be used in wounds. Other antiseptics, povidone-iodine, for example, have been used in wounds,[27] but their role in wound care has not been adequately studied.

RECOMMENDATIONS

1. Surveillance and Classification

a. 1) At the time of operation or shortly after, all operations should be classified and recorded as clean, clean-contaminated, contaminated, or dirty and infected (see text). *Category I*
   2) The classification should be recorded as such in the medical record. *Category II*

   b. The person in charge of surveillance of surgical patients should gather the information necessary to compute the classification-specific wound infection rates for all operations in the hospital. These rates should be computed at least every 6 to 12 months, entered into the records of the infection control committee, and made available to the department of surgery. *Category I*

   c. Every 6 to 12 months, procedure-specific clean wound infection rates should be computed for the hospital and all active surgeons. These rates should be given to all surgeons so that they can compare their own rate with that of others; the rates can be coded so that names do not appear. *Category II*

   d. An effort should be made to contact discharged patients to determine the infection rate for the 30 days after operation. *Category III*

2. Preparation of the Patient Before Operation

   a. If the operation is elective, all bacterial infections that are identified, excluding ones for which the operation is performed, should be treated and controlled before the operation. *Category I*

   b. The hospital stay before the operation should be as short as possible; in particular, tests and therapeutic measures that will prolong the preoperative stay beyond one day should be performed as outpatient services if possible. *Category III*

   c. If the operation is elective and the patient is grossly malnourished, the patient should receive oral or parenteral hyperalimentation before the operation. *Category II*

   d. If the operation is elective, the patient should bathe (or be bathed) the night before with an antiseptic soap. *Category III*

   e. **1)** Unless hair near the operative site is so thick that it will interfere with the surgical procedure, it should not be removed. *Category II*

       2) If hair removal is necessary, it should be done as near the time of operation as possible, preferably immediately before. *Category II*

    f. **1)** The area around and including the operative site should be scrubbed with a detergent solution followed by application of an antiseptic solution. This area should be large enough to include the entire incision and an adjacent area large enough for the surgeon to work during the operation without contacting unprepared skin. *Category I*

        2) Tincture of chlorhexidine, iodophors, and tincture of iodine are the recommended antiseptic products for preparing a patient's operative site. Plain soap, alcohol, or hexachlorophene are not recommended as single agents for operative site preparation unless the patient's skin is sensitive to the recommended antiseptic products. Aqueous quaternary ammonium compounds should not be used. *Category I*

    g. For major operations involving an incision and requiring use of the operating room (OR), the patient should be covered with sterile drapes in such a manner that no part of the patient is uncovered except the operative field and those parts necessary for anesthesia to be administered and maintained. *Category I*

3. Preparation of the Surgical Team

    a. Everyone who enters the OR should wear at all times 1) a high-efficiency mask to fully cover the mouth and nose; 2) a cap or hood to fully cover head hair; and 3) shoe covers.
        A beard should be fully covered by the mask and hood. *Category I*

    b. **1)** The surgical team (those who will touch the sterile surgical field, sterile instruments, or an incisional wound) should scrub their hands and arms to the elbows with an antiseptic before each operation. Scrubbing should be done before every procedure and take at least five minutes before the first procedure of the day. *Category I*

        2) Between consecutive operations, scrubbing times of two to five minutes may be acceptable. *Category III*

        3) Chlorhexidine, iodophors, and hexachlorophene are the recommended active antimicrobial ingredients for

the surgical hand scrub. Aqueous quaternary ammon-
ium compounds, for example, benzalkonium chloride,
should not be used. *Category I*

4) Hexachlorophene should not be used by pregnant
   women. *Category II*

c. 1) After the hands are scrubbed with an antiseptic and
      dried with a sterile towel, the surgical team should don
      sterile gowns. *Category I*

   2) Gowns used in the OR should be made of reusable or
      disposable fabrics that have been shown to be nearly
      impermeable to bacteria, even when wet. *Category II*

d. 1) The surgical team should wear sterile gloves. If a glove
      is punctured during the operation, it should be promptly
      changed. *Category I*

   2) For open bone operations and orthopedic implant
      operations, two pairs of sterile gloves should be worn.
      Category II

4. Ventilation and Air Quality in the Operating Room

a. All OR doors should be kept closed except as needed for
   passage of equipment, personnel, and the patient; personnel allowed to enter the OR, especially after an operation
   has started, should be kept to a minimum. *Category I*

b. For new construction, OR ventilation should include a
   minimum of 25 air changes per hour. All inlets for outside
   air should be located as high above ground as possible and
   remote from exhaust outlets of all types. All air, recircu-
   lated or fresh, should be filtered before entering the OR.
   Category I

5. Cleaning and Culturing in the OR and Culturing Personnel

a. The OR should be cleaned between surgical operations,
   daily, and weekly, according to established procedures for
   each scheduled cleaning. *Category I*

b. *Routine* culturing of the OR environment or personnel who
   use the OR should *not* be done (see Guidelines for Hospital

Environmental Control: Microbiologic Surveillance of the Environment and of Personnel in the Hospital). *Category I*

c. Use of tacky or antiseptic mats at the entrance to the OR is *not* recommended for infection control. *Category I*

6. Operative Technique

The surgical team should work in a manner such that the operation is performed as efficiently as possible in order to handle tissues gently, prevent bleeding, eradicate dead space, and minimize devitalized tissue and foreign material in the wound. *Category I*

7. Wound Care

a. Incisional wounds that are classified as "dirty and infected" should not ordinarily have skin closed over them at the end of an operation, that is, they should not ordinarily be closed primarily. *Category I* (If an operation is performed as part of the treatment of a low grade infection involving an implanted device, it is sometimes better to close the wound after operation to prevent superinfection with microorganisms more virulent than those already causing infection.)

b. If drainage is necessary for an uninfected wound, a closed suction drainage system should be used and placed in an adjacent stab wound rather than the main incisional wound. *Category I*

c. Personnel should wash their hands before and after taking care of a surgical wound. *Category I*

d. Personnel should not touch an open or fresh wound directly unless they are wearing sterile gloves. When the wound is sealed, dressings may be changed without gloves. *Category I*

e. Dressings over closed wounds should be removed if they are wet or if the patient has signs or symptoms suggestive of infection, for example, fever or unusual wound pain. When the dressing is removed, the wound should be inspected for signs of infection. Any drainage from a wound that is suspected of being infected should be cultured and smeared for Gram stain. *Category I*

8. Prophylactic Antibiotics, General Principles

a. Parenteral antibiotic prophylaxis is recommended for operations that 1) are associated with a high risk of infection, for example, most alimentary tract operations, cesarean sections, hysterectomies, and selected biliary tract operations; and 2) are not frequently associated with infection but, if infection occurs, are associated with severe or life-threatening consequences, for example, cardiovascular, neurosurgical, and orthopedic operations involving implantable devices. *Category I*

b. Except for cesarean sections, parenteral antibiotic prophylaxis should be started within two hours before the operation. These antibiotics should not be continued for more than 48 hours, although a 12-hour limit is desirable for most types of wounds and operations. *Category I* (For cesarean sections, prophylaxis is usually given intraoperatively after the umbilical cord is clamped.)

c. Oral, absorbable prophylactic antibiotics should not be used to supplement or extend parenteral prophylaxis. *Category I*

d. If oral antibiotics are used as prophylaxis with colo-rectal operations, their use should be limited to the 24 hours before the operation. *Category I*

e. Antibiotics selected for use as prophylaxis should have been shown to be effective for prophylaxis of operative wound infections in randomized, prospective, and controlled trials whose results have been published. *Category II*

f. Antibiotics given to patients whose wounds are classified as "dirty and infected" should be considered therapeutic rather than prophylactic. The antibiotic and its duration of use should be determined by clinical factors, for example, the pathogens likely to be involved, the site and severity of infection, and clinical response. *Category I*

9. Topical Antimicrobial Products

If used in the wound, topical antimicrobial products, either antibiotics or antiseptics, should be free of serious local or systemic side effects. *Category I*

REFERENCES

1. HALEY RW, HOOTON TM, CULVER DH, et al: Nosocomial infections in U.S. hospitals, 1975–1976: Estimated frequency by selected characteristics of patients. Am J Med 1981;70: 947–959.

2. CENTER FOR DISEASE CONTROL: Trends in surgical wound infection rates—United States. Morbid Mortal Weekly Rep 1980;29:27–28, 33.

3. HOWARD JM, BARKER WF, CULBERTSON WR, et al: Postoperative wound infections: The influence of ultraviolet irradiation of the operating room and various other factors. Ann Surg 1964;160(Suppl):1–192.

4. ALTEMEIER WA: Surgical infections: Incisional wounds. In: Bennett JV, Brachman PS (eds): *Hospital Infections.* Boston: Little, Brown and Company, 1979;287–306.

5. AMERICAN COLLEGE OF SURGEONS COMMITTEE ON CONTROL OF SURGICAL INFECTIONS: *Manual on Control of Infection in Surgical Patients.* Philadelphia, JB Lippincott: 1976.

6. CRUSE PJE, FOORD R: The epidemiology of wound infection. A ten-year prospective study of 62,939 wounds. Surg Clin North Am 1980;60:27–40.

7. ABER RC, GARNER JS: Postoperative wound infections. In: Wenzel RP (ed): *Handbook of Hospital Acquired Infections.* Boca Raton, Florida: CRC Press, Inc., 1981;303–316.

8. BRUUN J: Postoperative wound infection: Predisposing factors and the effect of a reduction in the dissemination of staphylococci. Acta Med Scand (suppl) 1970;514:(suppl) 1–89.

9. SEROPIAN R, REYNOLDS BM: Wound infections after preoperative depilatory versus razor preparation. Am J Surg 1971; 121:251–254.

10. DINEEN P: An evaluation of the duration of the surgical scrub. Surg Gynecol Obstet 1969;129:1181–1184.

11. GALLE PC, HOMESLEY HD, RHYNE AL: Reassessment of the surgical scrub. Surg Gynecol Obstet 1978;147:215–218.

12. WALTER CW, KUNDSIN RB: The bacteriologic study of surgical gloves from 250 operations. Surg Gynecol Obstet 1969;129:949–952.

13. U.S. DEPARTMENT OF HEALTH, EDUCATION, AND WELFARE: Minimum requirements of construction and equipment for

hospitals and medical facilities. (HRA 79-145000). Washington, DC: U.S. Government Printing Office, 1979.

14. MOGGIO M, GOLDNER L, McCOLLUM D, BEISSINGER S: Wound infections in patients undergoing total hip arthroplasty: Ultraviolet light for the control of airborne bacteria. Arch Surg 1979;114:815–823.

15. SCHWARTZ JT, SAUNDERS DE: Microbial penetration of surgical gown materials. Surg Gynecol Obstet 1980;150:507–512.

16. MOYLAN JA, KENNEDY BV: The importance of gown and drape barriers in the prevention of wound infection. Surg Gynecol Obstet 1980;151:465–470.

17. LAUFMAN H, EUDY WW, VANDERNOOT AM, LIU D, HARRIS CA: Strikethrough of moist contamination by woven and nonwoven surgical materials. Ann Surg 1975;181:857–862.

18. LANGE K: AORN standards for OR sanitation. AORN J 1975;21:1223–1231.

19. LAUFMAN H: Surgical hazard control: Effect of architecture and engineering. Arch Surg 1973;107:552–559.

20. McILRATH DC, VAN HEERDEN J, EDIS AJ: Closure of abdominal incisions with subcutaneous catheters. Surgery 1976;4:4112–4116.

21. van der LINDEN W, GEDDA S, EDLUND G: Randomized trial of drainage after cholecystectomy: Suction versus static drainage through a main wound versus a stab incision. Am J Surg 1981;141:289–294.

22. VERRIER ED, BOSSART KJ, HERR FW: Reduction of infection rates in abdominal incisions by delayed wound closure techniques. Am J Surg 1979;138:22–28.

23. POLK HC Jr, LOPEZ-MAYOR JF: Postoperative wound infection: A prospective study of determinant factors and prevention. Surgery 1969;66:97–103.

24. STONE HH, HANEY BB, KOLB LD, GEHEBER CE, HOOPER CA: Prophylactic and preventive antibiotic therapy: Timing, duration, and economics. Ann Surg 1979;189:691–699.

25. HURLEY DL, HOWARD P, HAHN HH II: Perioperative prophylactic antibiotics in abdominal surgery: A review of recent progress. Surg Clin North Am 1979;59:919–933.

26. MAKI DG: Lister revisited: Surgical antisepsis and asepsis. N Engl J Med 1976;294:1286–1287.

27. VILJANTO J: Disinfection of surgical wounds without inhibition of normal wound healing. Arch Surg 1980;115:253–256.

REFERENCE AUTHOR INDEX

An *f* following a page number represents a figure; a *t* indicates tabular material.

SUBJECT INDEX

An *f* following a page number represents a figure; a *t* indicates tabular material.

188